Reader's Digest

Complete A-Z of Medicine & Health

VOLUME ONE

Symptom sorter

Abdominal pain to Behaviour

Reader's Digest

Complete A-Z of Medicine & Health

VOLUME ONE

PUBLISHED BY THE READER'S DIGEST ASSOCIATION LIMITED
LONDON • NEW YORK • SYDNEY • MONTREAL

Contributors & Consultants

MEDICAL ADVISERS

Dr Sarah Brewer
MA MB BCHIR

Dr Alex Clarke
DPSYCH MSc BSc (HONS) AFBPsS

Dr John Cormack
BDS MB BS MRCS LRCP

Dr Vincent Forte
BA MB BS MRCGP MSc DA

Dr Judith Hall
BSc PHD MBPS

Dr Jim Lawrie
MB BS FRCGP MA (OXON) MBE

Sheena Meredith
MB BS MRCS (ENG) LRCP (LOND)

Dr Ian Morton
BSc PHD MIBIOL

Dr Melanie Wynne-Jones
MB CHB MRCGP DRCOG

CONTRIBUTORS

Elizabeth Adlam MA
Harriet Ainley BSc
Susan Aldridge MSc PhD
Dr Michael Apple BA
    MBChB MRCGP
Toni Battison RGN RSCN
    PgDip.
Glenda Baum MSc MCSP
    SRP
Nikki Bradford
Dr Sarah Brewer MA MB
    BChir
Pat Broad
Dr Harry Brown MBChB
    DRCOG MRCGP
Jenny Bryan BSc (Hons)
Rita Carter
Dr Alex Clarke DPsych MSc
    BSc (Hons) AFBPsS
Drew Clode BA
Geraldine Cooney BA
Dr John Cormack BDS MB
    BS MRCS LRCP
Dr Christine Fenn BSc
    (Hons) PhD
Dr Vincent Forte BA MB BS
    MRCGP MSc DA
Dr Judith Hall BSc PhD
    MBPS
William Harvey BSc (Hons)
    MCOptom
Caroline Holland BA
John Isitt BA
Dr Gillian Jenkins BM
    DRCOG DFFP BA
Georgina Kenyon BA
Dr Laurence Knott BSc
    (Hons) MB BS

Dr Jim Lawrie MBBS
    FRCGP MA (Oxon)
    MBE
Dr Patricia Macnair MA
    MBChB Dip Aneasth
Oona Mashta BA (Hons)
Sheena Meredith MB BS
    MRCS (Eng) LRCP
    (Lond)
Denise Mortimore BSc
    (Hons) PhD DHD
Dr Ian Morton BSc PhD
    MIBiol
John Newell MA (Camb)
Dr Louise Newson BSc
    (Hons) MB ChB (Hons)
    MRCP MRCGP
Nigel Perryman
Jim Pollard BA MA PCGE
Dr Ann Robinson MBBS
    MRCGP DCH DRCOG
Dr Christina Scott-Moncrieff
    MB ChB FFHom
Helen Spence BA
Dr Jenny Sutcliffe PhD MB
    BS MCSP
Jane Symons
June Thompson RN RM
    RGV
Helen Varley BA
Patsy Wescott BA (Hons)
Ann Whitehead MB BS
    MRCS LRCP MFFP
Dr Melanie Wynne-Jones
    MB ChB MRCGP
    DRCOG

CONSULTANTS & ORGANIZATIONS

Alcohol Concern

Alzheimer's Society

Dr Keith Andrews MD FRCP, The Royal Hospital for Neuro-disability

Arterial Disease Clinic

Association of British Insurers

Association for Postnatal Illness

BackCare

Toni Battison RGN RSCN PgDip

Blood Pressure Association

British Dental Health Foundation – Dr Nigel L. Carter BDS LDS (RCS)

British Dyslexia Association

British Lung Foundation

British Red Cross

Cancer Research UK

Candle Project – St Christopher's Hospice

Dr A Cann, University of Leicester

Chartered Institute of Environmental Health

CJD Support Network – Alzheimer's Society

Charles Collins MA ChM FRCS Ed – Member of Council for the Royal College of Surgeons of England

Dr Carol Cooper MA MB BChir MRCP

Cystic Fibrosis Trust

Mr R D Daniel BSc (Hons) FRCS FRCOphth DO

Mr Dai Davies FRCS (plas)

Department of Health – Public Awareness

Diabetes UK

Down's Syndrome Association

DrugScope

Eating Disorders Association

The Eyecare Trust

Family Planning Association

Food Standards Agency

Dr Vincent Forte BA MB BS MRCGP MSc DA

Professor Anthony Frew MA MD FRCP

Dr Judith Hall BSc PhD MBPS

International Glaucoma Association

Dr Rod Jaques DRCOG RCGP Dip. Sports Med. (Dist.)

Dr Laurence Knott BSc (Hons) MB BS

Dr Richard Long MD FRCP

Dr John Lucocq MB BCh BSc PhD

Mr W.A. Macleod MBChB FRCSE

Pamela Mason BSc PhD MRPharmS

ME Association

Meningitis Research Foundation

Migraine Action Association

Ian Morton BSc PhD MIBiol

Motor Neurone Disease Association

Multiple Sclerosis Society

National Addiction Centre

National Asthma Campaign

National Autistic Society

National Blood Service

National Eczema Society

National Hospital for Neurology and Neurosurgery

National Kidney Research Fund

National Society for the Prevention of Cruelty to Children

Pituitary Foundation

RADAR (The Royal Association for Disability and Rehabilitation)

RELATE

Dr Ann Robinson MBBS MRCGP DCH DRCOG

Royal College of Anaesthetists

Royal College of Speech and Language Therapists

Royal National Institute for Deaf People

Royal National Institute of the Blind

Royal Society for the Prevention of Accidents

Society for Endocrinology

The Society of Chiropodists and Podiatrists and Emma Supple FCPodS

SCOPE

Speakability

Penny Stanway MB BS

Terrence Higgins Trust

Dr Mark Westwood MA(Oxon) MRCP

Your family your

Good health is something we often take for granted. And rightly so: feeling well is our natural, normal state. We all want long life and well-being for ourselves, our families and our dependants.

But caring for your health can be a bewildering business. The language of medicine is difficult, the science is harder still, the complexity of the issues and the range of options available to patients are baffling. The aim of this encyclopedia is to help you to manage your health, to put you in a position where you can make clear and informed decisions about your treatment, your constitution, your life.

Many of the entries in the encyclopedia are descriptions of diseases or definitions of medical terms, including the wide range of complementary therapies now available. The information in these entries will help you to decide when to go to your doctor, what questions to ask when you are there, how to interpret the answers. If you are told that you have to undergo a medical procedure – say, a gastroscopy – then the encyclopedia will tell you what to expect and how to prepare for it. It also answers specific questions: what is the scientific basis for acupuncture? How do I get a referral to a cardiac specialist? Which is the best hearing aid for me? Throughout the seven A-Z volumes, you will find advice on such topics as guarding against high blood pressure, or living with Parkinson's disease. There is also information on big social and medical issues – drug addiction, care of the elderly, parenting – that we may all have to face.

To help you to find your way around the encyclopedia, there is an extensive index at the end of volume 7; within each article you will find cross-references along with lists of related topics at the end of the piece; a word in bold type means that there

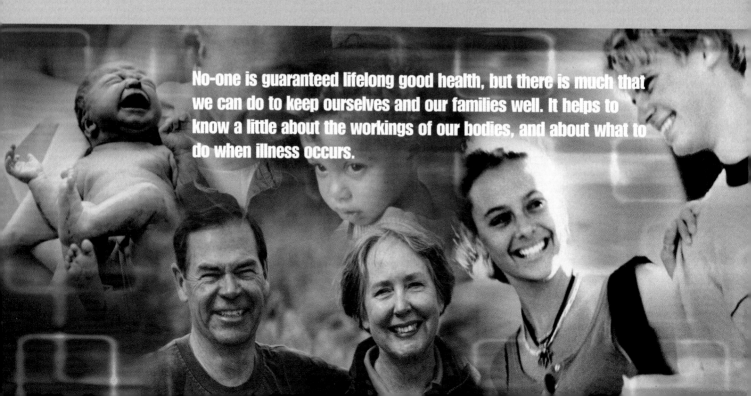

No-one is guaranteed lifelong good health, but there is much that we can do to keep ourselves and our families well. It helps to know a little about the workings of our bodies, and about what to do when illness occurs.

health

is a separate entry in the encyclopedia on that subject which you might like to consult. These devices will lead you through the pages, helping you to achieve the best possible understanding of any subject that concerns you.

Health and happiness

Good health is fundamental to human happiness. Through the ages, people have found that they can face almost any misfortune so long as they feel hale and strong. Conversely, chronic ill health can take the joy out of life, and make its smallest challenges appear insuperable.

So it is not surprising that, at every level of human activity, so much time and ingenuity is expended on the task of keeping people well and preventing disease. We all naturally try to safeguard our own health; pharmaceutics, the business of creating and marketing medicinal drugs, is a giant commercial venture worldwide; and of course all governments devote a huge proportion of their budgets to healthcare and health education.

Health in the UK

In Britain it has long been a source of national pride that the state provides healthcare free of charge to all citizens. This, at least, was the intention of the idealistic men and women who founded the National Health Service in the aftermath of the Second World War. In the half-century or so since then, the role of the NHS and the nature of our contact with it has changed. Prescriptions and dental care are no longer free – though they are still subsidised by the state. Hospitals and doctors' surgeries manage their own budgets, which affects the number and the nature of the services they provide. Additionally, there is a whole parallel structure of private medicine, which means that people can, if they wish,

'The sum of our medical knowledge has increased more in the past thirty years than in the preceding two hundred.'

pay to receive medical care more quickly, with more treatment options, and in more comfortable surroundings.

There is also a recognition that within the NHS some healthcare providers are better than others, either through a deliberate policy of specialization or simply because they are better organized or staffed. This has led the government to publish 'league tables' which allow patients to choose where they receive their care – just as they might choose to give their custom to one supermarket over another.

Medicine today

We hear a great deal about the shortcomings of British healthcare, but amid this criticism, it is easy to forget that we live in a golden age of medicine. The present generation can expect to live longer than any previous one. Most of us have access to sophisticated, up-to-date medicine when needed. Moreover, in the course of a 21st-century lifetime we can hope to experience less pain than our forebears, to avoid or survive more life-threatening conditions, and to have more control over and understanding of our health.

This is a time of constantly accelerating medical progress. There are treatments, tests and cures that were unheard of only a few years ago. This exponential rate of change no longer surprises us. We have lost sight of an astonishing fact – that the sum of medical knowledge has increased more in the past 200 years than in the previous 2000, and more in the past 30 than the previous 200. In the next 10 years the pace of discovery will be faster still.

The present medical revolution began around 1800 with the first experiments in vaccination. At that time doctors had no idea how disease was transmitted, or how to prevent it. It was Louis Pasteur who demonstrated that disease was caused by germs and bacteria which invade the body and multiply there. In the 1850s Ignaz Semmelweiss challenged the idea that deaths in childbirth were caused by bad air or 'hospital miasma'. He saved dozens of lives simply by insisting that doctors wash their hands between dissecting diseased bodies and entering the wards. Joseph Lister achieved a similar advance in surgery by pioneering the use of antiseptics and the sterilization of instruments.

The past hundred years is crowded with medical milestones. X-rays were discovered at the turn of the twentieth century – until then surgeons had no clear idea before they operated what they might find; aspirin, instant access to pain relief, became available at the same time; and penicillin, the first antibiotic, was discovered during the Second World War. The world's first heart transplant was performed in 1967 and the first 'test-tube baby' was born in 1978.

These last two events made headlines around the world at the time, but are now so commonplace as to be unremarkable. There have been many even more recent advances: keyhole techniques, which make surgery much less of a trauma than it used to be; the early detection and successful treatment of many cancers; and the huge improvement in the survival prospects for premature babies.

Ethical challenges

But in some areas progress is so rapid that there has not been time for us to discuss its wider implications. Our technical ability is racing ahead of the ethical debate. The present boom in genetics, for example, could mean that one day we might even be able to mould the characteristics of unborn children. But is it right to intervene in this way? Stem-cell research could lead to cures for conditions as diverse as diabetes and spinal-cord injuries, but in some countries this type of research is still the subject of intense controversy, particularly when embryonic stem cells are employed in the research procedures.

This ethical dimension does not just affect the outer reaches of medical research; it also concerns attitudes to everyday medical care. We are living through a fundamental shift in the doctor-patient relationship. Increasingly, it is seen as right and proper that we should be offered a range of treatment choices; that we – not the health professionals – should make the decisions about the medical procedures that we undergo; and that we have the right to challenge or criticise our healthcare providers. Some see this movement – one might call it 'patients' rights' – as a healthy dose of democracy for a traditionally authoritarian medical profession. Others think it is a mistake to cast the patient in the role of a consumer, because medicine is too complex and delicate a discipline to be governed by the blunt rules of the marketplace.

The rights of an individual patient can also conflict with the greater good of the community, and this is another area of hot debate. It includes the controversy over euthanasia (who decides when an individual life is not worth living?). It encompasses the care of the elderly (how do we manage the social and financial burden now that so many of us live to old age?). There are difficult issues about the right to opt out of state-sponsored vaccination programmes, and about the possibly catastrophic consequences of the overuse of antibiotics. All these questions will have to be addressed by doctors, politicians and society as a whole in the course of the next decade.

The triumph of technology and the new primacy of the patient have transformed medical practice. But our idea of medicine is also being deeply affected by the explosion of interest in complementary therapies. As recently as a generation ago, practices such as homeopathy, yoga and acupuncture were considered medical curiosities or, at worst, shameless quackery. But now there is a recognition that the traditional systems of Chinese and Indian medicine are rooted in profound philosophies of the body. Our growing understanding of this ancient thinking is helping to give us in the West a more rounded vision of the source of illness and the path to well-being. At the very least, most doctors would now accept that such therapies can be a useful adjunct to mainstream techniques – which is why they are now usually termed 'complementary' rather than 'alternative'.

All of these changes mean that we can be more self-aware and more self-reliant when it comes to our health. In today's world we often know – or we can find out – how best to remain well. And if we become ill, it is largely up to us to decide what to do about it.

This encyclopedia will help you to deal with that lifelong responsibility, to enjoy all the benefits of well-being. The essayist Izaak Walton wrote a wise thing 350 years ago. 'Look to your health; and if you have it, praise God,' he said. 'For health is a blessing that money cannot buy.'

'Not long ago, alternative practices such as homeopathy, yoga and acupuncture were looked on as medical curiosities or, at worst, shameless quackery.'

The human body is a truly marvellous machine. It is versatile, durable, capable of self-defence, and able to accomplish remarkable intellectual feats. And it requires – for most of a lifetime – relatively unsophisticated maintenance.

Though we are all individuals, different in detail, every human body is built to the same basic plan. The key to the way in which the body works lies in the fact that its various cells and organs are arranged into 'systems' (all of them described in detail in this encyclopedia). None of these systems works independently. The healthy functioning of each one depends on the smoothly co-ordinated performance of the others – not least the brain, which is the body's control centre. For this reason, total health demands that we attend to the needs of both body and mind.

Processing energy

Like any other living thing, the human body needs energy to stay alive, and it is superbly designed to extract the energy locked up in the food we eat. This process takes place in a cascade of reactions within the digestive system, which is essentially a bulging, twisted tube 7.5 metres long. As food enters the mouth and moves to the stomach, it is physically and chemically mashed into molecules small enough for the body to use. In the intestine the digestive and blood systems run so close together that food substances can pass into the blood for circulation to every part of the body. The solid wastes that remain are packaged and ejected from the end of the tube.

Meanwhile, food molecules travel to cells where they provide the energy to keep the whole organism alive and functioning. These food molecules are also the building blocks for cell maintenance and repair, and for the manufacture of vital control chemicals, notably the hormones. Some are stored for later use – but to make their energy available for movement or to keep the body warm, they need to be burned. Like the logs in a fireplace, the body's fuel needs oxygen to combust and release its energy. And oxygen is always on tap. It is obtained from the air through the tubes and bellows of the respiratory system; and it is supplied via blood pumped round the body by the tireless heart.

Minute by minute, the poisonous by-products of this energy generation are efficiently dealt with. Carbon dioxide, made when oxygen burns body fuels, is carried by the blood to the lungs from where it is exhaled. Chemical debris travels in the blood to the liver for processing and detoxification, then on to the kidneys and bladder for disposal.

'The body is superbly designed to extract the energy which is locked up in the food that we eat.'

The body systems

Fully supplied with energy, our bodies perform actions as different as running for a bus, or the minute manipulation that embroidery involves, or the contractions that keep the heart pumping for a lifetime.

Movement is effected through the action of the 206 bones in the skeletal system and through more than 600 muscles. The skeleton is made flexible by joints that articulate bone-on-bone. We move our limbs and turn our heads as muscles, attached to bones via tendons and ligaments, contract to manipulate joints. The joints are designed to enable a wide range of movements – 'ball and socket' joints at the shoulders and hips, hinge joints at the elbows and in the fingers.

Data management

Messages are constantly flashing round your body's communication network. When you want to stand up, for example, muscles and bones are responding to orders from the brain and nervous system, the body's central processor unit. When you speak you use muscles, including the large muscle that is the tongue, to mould air in the respiratory system in such a way that it creates speech. Though everyone is aware that they can control their actions like this, much of the operation of these systems goes on below the level of consciousness. Our brain and nervous

'Movement of the body is effected by the action of the 206 bones in the skeletal system and by more than 600 muscles.'

systems work unbidden to keep our lungs breathing and our digestive systems processing food. They regulate heartbeat, make the correct muscles contract to keep us standing upright. Through pain they signal when the body is threatened by injury or disease.

The brain and nervous system, like any operational HQ, can respond only on the basis of the information they receive. This is where the senses come in. Bombarding the brain is a huge mass of data from the outside world and from inside the body, too. Our eyes and ears provide information about the world around us; our ears also tell us how our bodies are oriented – for instance whether we are standing up or lying down. With the taste buds of the tongue and bulb-like receptors lining our noses we gather data in the form of taste and smell. Thanks to specialized nerve endings in the skin we can tell whether objects are hot or cold.

Information travels to and from the brain through myriad branches of the nervous system. The trunk route to and from the brain is the spinal cord. The nervous system sends its messages by means of tiny electrical signals, travelling at up to 250 mph, which are converted to chemical signals where nerve meets nerve. And the data contained in its messages are many and varied. They could signal that you recognize the face you just caught

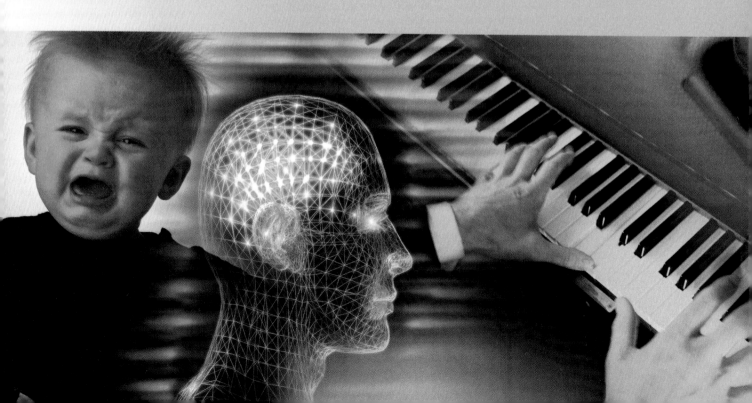

sight of; that you are hungry and need to find food fuel; that you are exercising, so your heart needs to beat faster and your lungs take in air more quickly.

The human brain is an evolutionary triumph. It gives us the power to think and feel, to have memories, to build cities and computers, to explore our world, to read and to write. Like other body systems, the brain is organized into different areas that have different functions. The cerebrum is the part of the brain responsible for our intelligence and mental skills. It is here that information from the senses is received and appreciated at an intellectual level.

Other parts of the brain specialize in storing and retrieving memories, and in controlling activities such as sleep. At a lower level, the central nervous system acts as a monitoring service for the body, managing reflex actions such as blinking, which keep the body in good shape and out of danger. If you step on a sharp stone it is a reflex nerve action, working via the spinal cord and bypassing the brain, that makes you pull your foot away.

Command and control

The brain and nervous system are the body's rapid-reaction control system, but they are not the body's only information providers. Many of the functions that need to take place without our conscious intervention are run by the hormonal or endocrine system. Hormones are released into the bloodstream, the body's fluid communication network. They are carried to all parts of the body, where they trigger such processes as the production of the hormones that control a child's growth.

In overall control of the endocrine system is the pituitary gland. The pituitary is the foreman in the hormonal factory. It oversees the production of other hormones including, for example, the wide range of sex hormones and also the thyroid hormones which control the metabolism. In its turn, the pituitary is managed by the hypothalamus, an outgrowth from the base of the brain. This close link between brain and hormones explains in part why the emotions have a powerful effect on the body. Fear of pregnancy, for instance, can disrupt the production of the hormones that control the release of eggs from a woman's ovaries.

Most hormones take time to exert their effects – a consequence of the fact that they travel in the blood. But one part of the hormonal system is fast-acting. When we are stressed, in pain, or frightened the glands that sit atop each kidney produce the hormones adrenalin and noradrenaline. These chemicals quickly prepare the body for 'fight or flight'. They make the heart beat faster, raise the blood pressure, speed up breathing and mobilize energy stores.

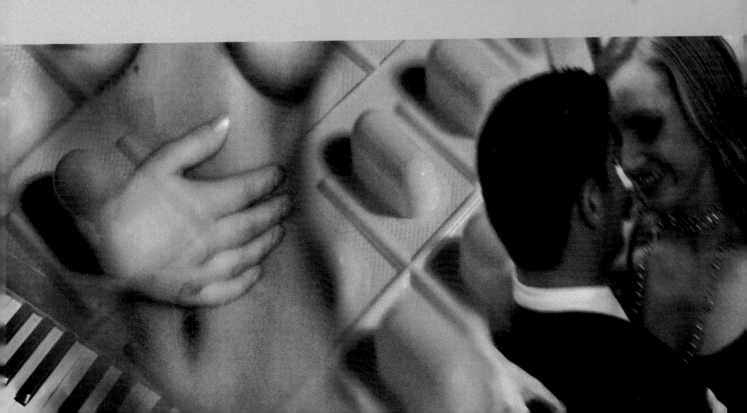

The systems that control hunger, thirst and body temperature are also vital to the upkeep of the human machine. The body is 70 per cent water, but we constantly lose it through the pores of our skin as we sweat (a process essential to controlling body temperature). We need to drink to keep supplies replenished, and we have a thirst control mechanism to make sure we do. It resides in the hypothalamus along with our 'appestat', the mechanism that sets off our internal hunger alarm. When the body is in need of water or food we are literally driven to find what we need. Yet the higher centres of the brain can override these basic survival mechanisms: we can eat when we are not hungry, or ignore hunger and go without if need be.

Protection and defence

Within and without, the body is armed with a surprising array of physical and chemical defences. The bones of the skull guard our brains from damage, the vertebrae are armour-plating for the spinal cord, our ribs encase our lungs like a protective cage, our hips provide a bony surround for the bladder.

The skin resists assault by countless micro-organisms and chemical molecules thanks in part to a thin covering of oil produced by glands within its layers. The skin also has an ability to counter the harmful effects of ultra-violet rays by producing the dark pigment melanin when exposed to sunshine. Minute hairs in our nostrils filter the air of potential invaders while sensory receptors in the skin respond to the dangers of heat, cold and pain.

There are also internal lines of defence, such as the ability of the blood to clot when a blood vessel is severed, and of scar tissue to grow over wounds. Deeper still, bones will re-knit when broken, and many organs – notably the liver – have the power to regenerate themselves to some degree. But of all the body's hidden defence forces, the most remarkable is the immune system. It operates largely through white blood cells (as opposed to the red blood cells that carry oxygen around the system). Its specialized cells are able to recognize when 'foreign' material has entered the body – usually bacteria or viruses – and to set in train a series of reactions to eliminate the invaders.

As part of this reaction, the body makes antibodies, molecules able to disrupt and disable intruders. And if we do succumb to the illness the invaders provoke, the production of antibodies is retained as a kind of chemical memory, giving immunity to subsequent onslaught by the same attackers.

The downside of the system is that the immune system immediately recognizes as 'foreign' tissue such as a skin or bone graft

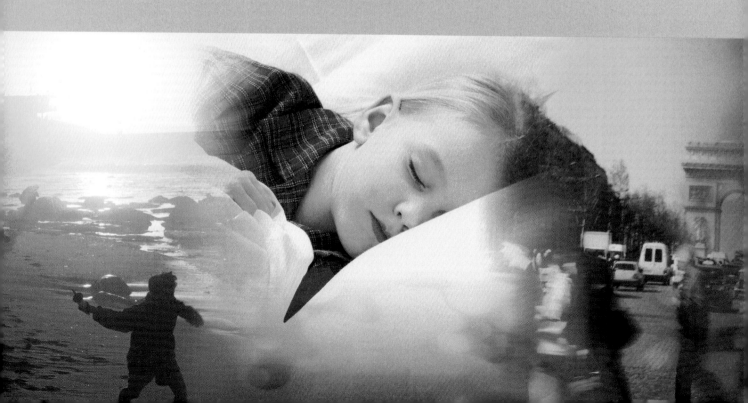

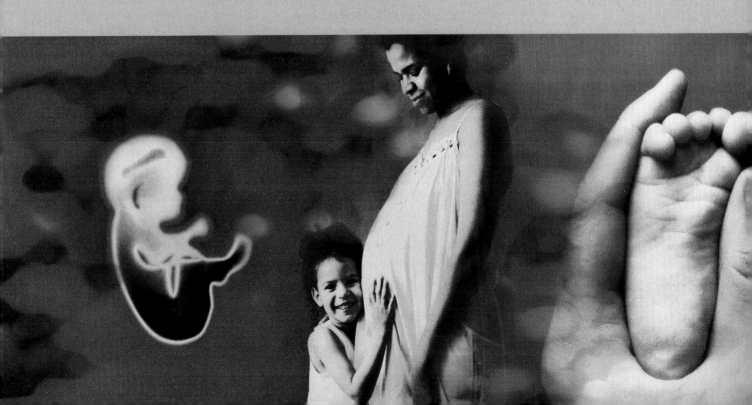

from another person. Only with the introduction of anti-immune drugs has it been possible for organ and tissue grafting to become successful.

A new generation

Like all living things, from the simplest amoeba upwards, we have the ability to reproduce ourselves. The basic elements of the male and female reproductive systems are present in boy and girl babies at birth. But they start to mature only at puberty largely as the result of hormonal controls directed by the pituitary gland.

Every 28 days or so, from puberty to menopause, a woman's ovaries release an egg and the lining of the uterus is prepared to receive and nourish it should it be fertilized. Unlike the cyclical on-off nature of the female reproductive system, the male system is designed so that it can go into action at a moment's notice. Sperm are produced continuously from puberty right up to old age: men can father children well into their eighties – and they sometimes do.

The male reproductive system is designed solely for sperm production and delivery, but the female system is more complex. As well as producing eggs and releasing them into an environment conducive to sperm, it must provide a secure place (the uterus) in which an

'Our genetic blueprint makes each one of us an unrepeatable exemplar of the same human template.'

embryo can become implanted, be nourished, and grow to full term. After birth a woman's breasts make milk which provides perfect nutrition for at least the first six months of a child's life.

As children grow and develop it quickly becomes obvious that each one is unique. Even identical twins, though they share the same genetic make-up, will form their own distinct personalities. This uniqueness derives ultimately from the most essential body 'system': the one that determines the individual nature of our genes. It is the genes which control the development and working of all the body parts. Our genetic blueprint has evolved over millions of years to make us the one-off sentient beings that we are: unrepeatable exemplars of the same human template.

However conscious we are of good health, and even if we do everything we can to maintain our body systems and keep them in tip-top condition, it is inevitable that our bodies eventually fail us. Cells and organs age, our immune systems wear out, or we are struck down by an accident.

Modern medicine is equipped as never before to compensate for the inefficiencies and inadequacies of the human frame. We will never find a cure for ageing, but research is beginning to unravel some of its secrets. In the meantime, there is much at which to marvel in the resilience and longevity of the human machine.

Symptom sorter

Symptoms are the sign that something is wrong somewhere in the body or mind. Knowing how to understand and evaluate your symptoms will help you to get the right treatment at the right time.

Contents

16–21   General symptoms

22–24   Chest problems

25–33   Skin and hair

34–37   Arms and legs, hands and feet

38–44   Head, face and neck

45–50   Stomach, bowel and abdomen

51–56   Female problems

57–59   Male problems

60–61   Urinary problems

62–63   Quick reference

The symptom sorter is not a tool for self-diagnosis and cannot replace objective professional medical assessment.

Every care has been taken to ensure that the information is up to date and accurate. It is a guide to understanding what symptoms might represent and what appropriate action to take. It has been thoroughly researched and is based on the everyday working experience and knowledge of practising NHS GPs. If you are in any doubt about the importance or urgency of a medical problem, always get advice from your NHS GP's surgery or go to your local hospital casualty department.

The Symptom sorter is designed to help you to make sense of the most common symptoms and to guide you to appropriate help. It covers the most common symptoms and their likely causes. The Quick reference on pages 62 and 63 includes other important symptoms, with advice on the action you should take for each.

How does the Symptom sorter work?

Within each section you will find each symptom discussed briefly in an introduction. The Symptom sorter will help you to interpret these symptoms. The most common causes are then discussed in the column headed Common causes. Next to this you will find information on Action, which tells you what to do and how quickly to do it.

You will also find a list of occasional and rare causes. It is important to be aware of these, but remember that they are much less likely to be the cause of that symptom than the common causes listed. Every symptom, no matter how ordinary it seems, has potentially serious causes. The Symptom sorter is a guide only, not a substitute for actual medical advice or management.

Over-the-counter remedies

For some symptoms the Action column advises using over-the-counter (OTC) remedies – retail products available from pharmacies without a GP's prescription. Always seek the pharmacist's advice when buying any OTC product and read the manufacturer's leaflet for contra-indications. Check with your GP if you are in any doubt.

Recommended action

The advice given in the Action column classifies levels of urgency as follows.
- **Dial 999**: in life-threatening emergencies, call an ambulance. Follow the instructions given by the operator and provide information as requested. Remain calm and speak clearly.
- **See GP urgently**: ask for an appointment that same day. If all appointments are already taken for that day, ask to speak to a GP to check how urgently you should be seen. All GPs in the UK provide a 24-hour service for medical emergencies. Outside of office hours most surgeries provide instructions on what to do in an answering message on their usual phone number. Alternatively, call NHS Direct (0845 4647); this will put you into contact with an experienced nurse who can advise you further.
- **See GP as soon as possible**: ask for the next available routine appointment. Most surgeries will be able to offer a space within a week or so.
- **See GP non-urgently**: ask for a routine appointment in the next few weeks or so.
- **Consult a genito-urinary medical clinic, drug and alcohol agency, counselling service**: you can arrange an appointment yourself without being referred by a doctor. To find local branches, consult the telephone directory or phone your local surgery or hospital.

Home visits

Doctors' home visits are generally reserved for people who are too ill to travel or whose medical condition would be made worse by a journey, for instance, those who are bedridden or dying, and people unable to walk more than a few yards. Doctors will not usually make home visits solely because a patient has difficulty in arranging travel.

In general, children, even those with fevers or who are vomiting, can be brought to a surgery. Your child may be seen more quickly this way than if you wait for a home visit.

Think before you request a home visit. Most GPs can see three or four patients in the time it takes to see just one patient at home.

First aid

For emergency treatment refer to the FIRST AID book.

1. Look at the symptom profile. This heading tells you which symptom is covered.

2. Move on to the second column for a list of the most common causes of each symptom.

3. Read the Action column to find out what to do and how urgently to do it.

Bruising

A brief description of the symptom explains its characteristics to help you to identify your problem.

Bruising is reddish-purple skin discoloration that does not whiten under pressure. The medical name is purpura.

Occasional and rare causes are listed alongside more likely causes. Main articles on most of these conditions can be found elsewhere in the encyclopedia.

OCCASIONAL CAUSES: painful bruising syndrome; connective tissue disorders (eg lupus erythematosis); vasculitis (inflammation of blood vessel walls); platelet (blood) defects; lichen sclerosus et atrophicus (a skin disease).
RARE CAUSES: bone marrow damage (caused by cytotoxic drugs, leukaemia or cancer); inherited blood-clotting disorders (eg, haemophilia); infections (eg, meningococcal septicaemia); deficiency of vitamin C or K .

COMMON CAUSES	ACTION
Injury Bruises can be any size, and are usually tender to the touch. The original injury is often minor. **Bruising**	No treatment needed, but cold compresses reduce swelling and arnica cream may help to speed up recovery. If repeated bruising appears on areas not subjected to everyday knocks, see GP as soon as possible.
Senile purpura (age-related bruising) Bruises often appear repeatedly, are widespread and without obvious cause. This is caused by fragile blood vessels in ageing skin.	See GP as soon as possible if there is unexplained bleeding of any sort as well; otherwise no action needed.
Liver disease (especially alcoholic cirrhosis) Widespread bruises of all sizes repeatedly appear. There may be other signs of liver disease or alcohol excess. **Liver disease**	See GP urgently: there may be a blood-clotting problem.
Coughing or vomiting Tiny bruises appear on the face immediately after a violent coughing fit or vomiting, which increases pressure in major blood vessels. Also seen inside lips and eyelids.	No action needed: it looks alarming but is of no importance in itself.
Drug reactions Widespread tiny bruises appear suddenly. They are not painful, but you may feel unwell from some other side effect of the drug (eg, steroids, aspirin, warfarin, quinine, thiazides).	See GP as soon as possible; urgently if you are taking warfarin.

The advice given here explains how to relieve your symptom, if appropriate, and whether to consult a doctor as an emergency or non-emergency.

Photographs help you to identify possible causes of symptoms.

The Common causes section lists the main conditions. Each entry has a brief description that explains how you might feel or look and any other associated factors that may be important.

Ten symptoms you should not ignore

Always consult a doctor urgently if you, or anyone in your care, has any of the following symptoms.

- Sudden, severe, crushing chest pain.
- Severe breathlessness.
- Sudden and lasting confusion or loss of consciousness.
- Severe headache and neck stiffness, particularly if associated with eye pain on looking at a normal-strength light.

- Sudden loss of vision.
- Severe and constant abdominal pain.
- Vomiting blood.
- Jet-black bowel motions.
- Diarrhoea and vomiting lasting more than 24 hours.
- Severe back pain with pain or numbness down both legs and sudden incontinence.

Symptom sorter

Glands, swollen

Swollen glands are enlarged lymph nodes – they swell and become noticeable when they are fighting infection, and may also be sore. The glands most easily felt are under the jaw, all around the neck and in the armpits and groin.

OCCASIONAL CAUSES: glandular fever; cat-scratch fever (common in children); sarcoidosis; German measles (rubella); measles; systemic lupus (an autoimuune inflammatory disease); rheumatoid arthritis; sexually transmitted diseases (eg lymphogranuloma venereum).

RARE CAUSES: AIDS and AIDS-related complex; tuberculosis; tropical diseases (eg leprosy); drug reactions.

COMMON CAUSES	ACTION
General viral infection This is the cause of nine out of ten cases of swollen glands. Enlarged glands may be felt around the body (in the neck, armpits, groin). You may be generally unwell, with a fever.	Rest, drink plenty of non-alcoholic fluids, take paracetamol regularly. If not beginning to improve after five days, call GP for advice.
Localized infection Enlargement of a single group of glands (such as in the neck). Fever and feeling generally unwell; possibly with specific symptoms such as cough or sore throat.	As for General viral infection, above.
Cancer Slowly enlarging, often painless, hard, fixed glands, usually in a single group. Present for six weeks or more.	See GP as soon as possible.
White cell cancers (lymphoma, leukaemia, myeloma) As for Cancer above, but may involve several groups of glands. Night sweats and itching common.	See GP as soon as possible.
Septicaemia (bacterial infection in bloodstream) Several groups of glands are enlarged. Feeling very ill, high fever; possible confusion and delirium.	Urgent GP assessment. A home visit may be necessary if you are confused.

Insomnia

Sleep needs vary with age and according to the individual: infants require at least 16 hours, while adults need 5–8 hours, some 3–4 hours. Insomnia should not be confused with a low requirement for sleep.

OCCASIONAL CAUSES: respiratory problems (eg asthma, chronic obstructive pulmonary disease); inefficient heart pumping (left ventricular failure); overactive thyroid (hyper-thyroidism); benzodiazepine withdrawal; parasomnias (eg nightmares, night terrors, sleepwalking); disruption of biorhythms (eg due to jet lag, shift work).

RARE CAUSES: malnutrition, low weight; post-traumatic stress disorder; mania; sleep apnoea (cessation of breathing in sleep).

COMMON CAUSES	ACTION
Excess psychological stress You are slow to go off to sleep, may have early morning waking, and feel low or nervous. (Underlying causes include problems with work, relationships or finances.)	See GP as soon as possible.
Clinical depression Early morning waking and low mood, along with low self-esteem, lack of confidence, poor short-term memory, tearfulness, irrational sense of guilt and other symptoms.	See GP as soon as possible.
Chronic excess alcohol Sleep may be totally disrupted. Other signs of alcohol abuse, such as red face and palms, are common.	Seek help from local drugs and alcohol agency.
Hyperstimulation (poor sleeping patterns) You may be wide awake at night and slow to go off, but otherwise well. (Caffeine and nicotine are common underlying causes.)	Change lifestyle to reduce stimulation at night.
Pain of chronic illness Sleep may be totally disrupted. The underlying cause, for example, osteoarthritis, is usually obvious.	See GP as soon as possible to deal with cause.

Libido, loss of

Loss of libido is loss of sex drive, and may be partial or total. The strength of libido may be reduced for some or all of the time, or it may be as strong but less frequent. Libido varies greatly between individuals; some people have naturally low libido.

OCCASIONAL CAUSES: ageing; anti-androgenic drugs that block testosterone; in men, antihypertensive treatment, drugs that increase prolactin (eg spironolactone, cimetidine). **RARE CAUSES:** pituitary or hypothalamic disease; testicular disease or damage; adrenal gland or kidney disease; in men, feminizing tumours in the testis or adrenal gland.

COMMON CAUSES	ACTION
Depression Low mood, tearfulness, loss of interest in pleasurable activities; loss of appetite, concentration and short-term memory; disrupted sleep and extreme fatigue.	If symptoms are present for two weeks or more, see GP as soon as possible.
Relationship problem Difficulties in relationship with partner, but no other problems.	Seek help from a counselling service, such as Relate.
Menopause Hot flushes, night sweats, mood swings, dry vagina, headaches and depression.	See GP non-urgently for assessment.
Excess alcohol intake (and cirrhosis in men) Signs of alcohol misuse such as lifestyle factors (eg spending too much time in the pub), red face and palms.	Reduce or stop drinking. Seek help from local drugs and alcohol agency. See GP non-urgently for checkup.
Underactive thyroid (hypothyroidism) Feeling cold, tired and slowed down. Hair brittle and skin dry. Weight gain is common.	See GP non-urgently for assessment.

Lightheadedness

Lightheadedness is a vague term that describes a sensation of giddiness, dizziness and feeling faint. There is often a sense of unreality or momentary confusion, but no loss of consciousness or actual fainting. It is not the same as vertigo, in which there is a sensation of the surroundings spinning around. It is a common feature of many medical problems.

OCCASIONAL CAUSES: acute drug and/or alcohol intoxication, chronic alcohol abuse; change in heart rhythm (cardiac arrhythmia); drug treatment (eg anti-hypertensives, anti-depressants); any serious disease. **RARE CAUSES:** narrowing of heart valve (aortic stenosis); blockage of the arteries; temporal lobe epilepsy and/or tumour; carbon monoxide poisoning.

COMMON CAUSES	ACTION
Viral infection Generally feeling unwell; fever usually present. Other possible symptoms include sore throat, cough, diarrhoea.	Rest, drink plenty of fluids, take paracetamol regularly. If it lasts over a week, see GP as soon as possible.
Low blood sugar (reactive hypoglycaemia) Sudden onset, usually 4–6 hours after a meal when rushing. Clammy sweatiness, weak feeling in body, irritable mood.	Take sugary drink and eat a biscuit or piece of bread. Glucose sweets may also help.
Low blood pressure (postural hypotension) Sudden lightheadedness on standing from sitting or lying. More common after a hot bath or in hot weather. May be caused by some medications (eg some antidepressants). Common in pregnant women and elderly people.	Lie down, preferably with feet higher than head, get up gradually after symptom has passed. See GP non-urgently if persistent.
Vertebro-basilar insufficiency Sudden onset on turning head in a particular direction, caused by reduced blood flow. Common in elderly people with osteoarthritis in the bones of the neck.	No specific treatment; avoid movement that triggers the problem. See GP non-urgently for diagnosis and advice.
Anxiety Fast breathing rate without exertion. Feelings of panic, tingling around mouth, in fingers and toes. If severe, hands and feet may develop cramps.	Calm symptoms: hold a paper bag loosely around your mouth and nose and breathe deeply. See GP non-urgently for advice.

Symptom sorter

Memory loss

Memory is classed as short-term (immediate), medium-term (recent) and long-term (remote). For memory loss with acute confusion, see page 62.

OCCASIONAL CAUSES: vitamin B₁ (thiamin) deficiency; artery disease; brain tumour. RARE CAUSES: subarachnoid haemorrhage (bleeding in brain); some personality disorders; very severe epilepsy; carbon monoxide poisoning; viral encephalitis (inflammation of the brain).

COMMON CAUSES	ACTION
Head injury A head injury can cause all levels of memory loss. If the injury is severe enough to affect the memory, hospitalization is usually needed.	Seek specialist advice from hospital team involved in initial care, or see a GP non-urgently if later.
Dementia, including Alzheimer's disease Gradual onset over a year or two. Short- and medium-term memory affected, long-term memory usually intact. Person usually unaware of problem.	See GP non-urgently for assessment and possible specialist referral.
Stroke Sudden onset. May be associated with collapse, weakness or loss of power of speech.	See GP urgently; a home visit may be necessary.
Depressive illness Gradual onset over two or more weeks, with loss of concentration, constant low mood; loss of appetite, self-esteem; sleep disturbance, fatigue. Usually aware of problem.	See GP as soon as possible for assessment.
Chronic excess alcohol intake Gradual onset. Signs of chronic alcohol excess (eg, lifestyle factors, red face and palms). Person often unaware of problem; invents stories to cover gaps in memory.	See GP as soon as possible. Requires careful assessment.

Muscles, painful

Pain in muscles may be experienced as a short-lived cramp, as a continuous dull ache or as a sharp and severe pain on using the affected muscle. It may be painful to touch as well as to use.

OCCASIONAL CAUSES: peripheral vascular disease (narrowing of blood vessels in legs and arms); diabetic or alcoholic neuropathy (nerve disease); general anaesthesia, side effect of muscle-relaxant drug; underactive thyroid (hypothyroidism); Bornholm disease (devil's grip). RARE CAUSES: side effect of drug treatment (eg chemotherapy, cimetidine) or drug withdrawal.

COMMON CAUSES	ACTION
Overuse of muscles, including strain Sudden onset after unusually intense or prolonged activity. Muscle sore to touch and stiff after rest.	Take OTC painkillers, apply heat rubs or take anti-inflammatories. Stay active without straining the affected muscle.
Acute viral illness Sudden onset, with fever and feeling generally unwell. Many muscles are affected, and pain may move from one area to another.	Rest, take non-alcoholic drinks, regular paracetamol or OTC anti-inflammatories. If not settling within five days, call GP for advice.
Depression, ME (myalgic encephalomyelitis)/ chronic fatigue syndrome Vague pains in many different muscles, usually worse after activity. Associated with low mood and tiredness.	See GP non-urgently for assessment.
Inflammatory myopathy (muscle disease) May start suddenly. Marked morning stiffness. Persistent, affecting specific muscles, which may be painful to touch. (Causes include rheumatoid arthritis and scleroderma.)	See GP urgently as some conditions are associated with serious complications if not treated.
Referred joint pain Pain associated with a nearby joint problem and referred (for example, from hip to thigh or shoulder to arm). Made worse if the affected joint is used then rested.	Take OTC painkillers and anti-inflammatories. See GP as soon as possible for assessment.

Numbness and pins and needles

Loss of feeling (numbness) and prickling (pins and needles) in the skin are known medically as paraesthesia. Commonly produced by sitting too long in one position, they may be accompanied by feelings of hot or cold and pain on light touch.

OCCASIONAL CAUSES: multiple sclerosis; spinal cord inflammatory disease (dorsal myelitis); alcoholic polyneuropathy (nerve disease) and vitamin B_1, B_6, and B_{12} deficiency; stroke; injury to peripheral nerve or spinal cord; low blood calcium (hypocalcaemia); kidney failure; low blood sugar (hypoglycaemia); porphyria (an enzyme deficiency); xanthomatosis (fatty deposits affecting nerves); Raynaud's syndrome.
RARE CAUSES: spinal cord tumour; brain trauma, tumour or epilepsy affecting sensory cortex; migraine.

COMMON CAUSES	ACTION
Anxiety with hyperventilation Nervous emotional state, episodes of dizziness, rapid breathing. Often affects hands, feet and area around mouth. In severe hyperventilation, feet and hands may spasm.	To calm symptoms, breathe in and out of a paper bag held loosely over mouth and nose. If not settling, call GP urgently for advice; otherwise see GP non-urgently for help.
Carpal tunnel syndrome (trapped nerve) Pins and needles, pain in hands. Worse at night and after manual work. Finger-thumb grip may be weak.	See GP as soon as possible for assessment.
Sciatica (spinal nerve root compression) Follows severe, sudden lower back pain: numbness and pain spreads from lower back through buttock and down back of leg to side of foot.	See GP urgently or ask for home visit. Try OTC painkillers. If both legs are affected, go straight to casualty: you may need to be hospitalized.
Diabetic neuropathy (nerve disease) Often continuous pins and needles; hot and cold sensations, pain. Affects one or more limbs.	See GP as soon as possible for assessment.
Arthritis in neck (cervical spondylosis) Pain and tingling in back, neck and top of head. Made worse by certain movements.	Take OTC anti-inflammatories or painkillers. If severe, see GP as soon as possible.

Sweating, excessive

Indications that sweating may be excessive are the clothes becoming soaked through, the forehead being constantly wet or the hands being constantly slippery. Excessive sweating may occur with or without heat.

OCCASIONAL CAUSES: drugs, including some antidepressants; alcohol and alcohol withdrawal; shock (eg a drop in blood pressure from haemorrhage); fainting; intense pain; palmar and plantar hyperhidrosis (excessive sweating from the palms and soles of the feet).
RARE: nerve damage (eg brain tumours, spinal cord injury); excess hormone production (eg caused by hyperpituitarism/acromegaly).

COMMON CAUSES	ACTION
Menopause Marked heat, skin flushing, and sudden drenching sweat, often worse at night. Possible mood swings, light and infrequent periods, vaginal dryness.	See GP non-urgently to discuss treatment of flushes alone or hormone replacement therapy (HRT) if suitable.
Anxiety Sweating may be sudden and related to a stressful event, or long-term as part of a chronic anxiety problem. Often also with shakiness of hands and clammy, cool skin.	Long-term anxiety can be helped by medication and psychological treatments. See GP non-urgently.
Infections Skin may also be hot or clammy, fever usually present. Feeling generally unwell, possible cough, pain passing urine.	See GP urgently for examination and treatment.
Low blood sugar (hypoglycaemia) Sudden sweating, clamminess, weak feeling, irritable mood. In non-diabetics, usually occurs 4–6 hours after a meal when rushing around; in diabetics, if a meal is missed.	Take sugary drink, biscuit or bread. If frequent, diabetics should review their drug dosing as soon as possible with GP.
Overactive thryroid (hyperthyroidism) Gradually feeling unwell, weight loss, shakiness of hands, fast pulse rate and sense of anxiety.	See GP as soon as possible for diagnosis (blood test) and treatment.

Symptom sorter

Tired all the time

This is the constant feeling of being tired and worn out. Physical and mental activities take more effort than usual, and the ability to keep going is reduced.

OCCASIONAL CAUSES:
ME (myalgic encephalitis) or chronic post-viral fatigue syndrome; major organ failure (eg heart, liver, kidney); overactive thyroid (hyperthyroidism); substance misuse; drugs (eg beta-blockers, diuretics).
RARE CAUSES: cancer; tuberculosis or other chronic infection; chronic neurological (nerve) disorders; diabetes mellitus, Addison's disease or other endocrine gland disorders; connective tissue disorders (eg rheumatoid arthritis, polymyalgia rheumatica).

COMMON CAUSES	ACTION
Depressive illness May be worse at some times of the day than others. Associated with tearfulness and loss of confidence, concentration, pleasure, self-esteem. Poor sleep.	If symptoms are present for two weeks or more, see GP as soon as possible. Should respond to treatment.
Stress Tiredness reduces when cause of stress is not present. Identifiable trigger: life circumstances such as overwork, young children or boredom.	Try relaxation tapes, yoga, exercise. Take time for self. See GP if this fails.
Anaemia (low red blood cell content) Constant tiredness. Pale lips, tongue and inner eyelids; in extreme cases, shortness of breath on exertion and fainting. Blood loss (for instance, heavy periods), or lack of iron or B vitamins (poor diet).	See GP as soon as possible, urgently if extreme symptoms are present.
Acute post-viral fatigue Recent illness. Constant, debilitating fatigue.	Rest, eat well. See GP if symptoms persist longer than a month after trigger illness.
Underactive thyroid (hypothyroidism) Gradual onset of constant, debilitating fatigue, associated with coldness and feeling slowed down. Skin may feel dry, hair brittle.	See GP as soon as possible for assessment and possible blood test.

Tremor

Tremor, a repetitive shaking movement of part of the body, is caused by rapid contraction and relaxation of the muscles. It is often noticed in the hands, but can affect any part of the body. It is often embarrassing for the person affected, and can interfere with everyday physical activity.

OCCASIONAL CAUSES:
adverse drug reaction; carbon dioxide retention in chronic obstructive pulmonary (lung) disease; multiple sclerosis; chronic liver disease ('liver flap', also called asterixis); any cause of ataxia (clumsy movement), eg tumour, abscess.
RARE CAUSES: hepatic encephalopathy (brain poisoning caused by liver malfunction).

COMMON CAUSES	ACTION
Anxiety Fast, racing heartbeat, palpitations. Nervous emotional state; life stresses likely. Sweaty skin, shaky hands; often breathlessness and pins and needles.	Consider ways to reduce life stress. See GP as soon as possible for confirmation and help.
Thyrotoxicosis (overactive thyroid) Consistently fast heartbeat with missed beats. Gradual, relentless weight loss; feeling hot and dislike of warm environments. Fine tremor of hands.	See GP as soon as possible for assessment.
Drug and alcohol withdrawal Sudden onset with confusion, generalized shaking, fast heartbeat and profuse sweating.	Risk of fits; contact GP urgently. If delirious and confused, dial 999.
Benign essential tremor Usually runs in families. Sufferers notice tremor disappears at rest or on taking alcohol. Otherwise well. Harmless, no known cause.	See GP non-urgently.
Parkinson's disease Tremor worst at rest. Slow movements, shuffling gait, frequent falls and inexpressive, mask-like face.	See GP as soon as possible.

Weight gain, excessive

Excessive weight gain is when your body weight is greater than it should be for your height and gender. This can be scientifically determined using the Body Mass Index (BMI): Weight (in kilograms) divided by Height (in metres)^2. A normal BMI is between 20 and 25. More than 30 is moderately overweight, and more than 40 is obese.

OCCASIONAL CAUSES: liver or kidney failure; drugs (eg steroids, insulin, sulphonylureas for diabetes, oestrogen); polycystic ovary syndrome (a hormonal disorder); mental retardation (eg Down's syndrome); physical disability restricting activity.
RARE CAUSES: anabolic steroid abuse; Cushing's syndrome (an adrenal disease); rare genetic syndromes (eg Prader-Willi).

COMMON CAUSES	ACTION
Simple obesity In men, fat tends to accumulate on the trunk; in women, on the breasts, bottom, hips, thighs. Ankle swelling possible in severe cases. No other symptoms.	Calorie-controlled diet, increased exercise. If this fails over a six-month period, see GP non-urgently.
Underactive thyroid (hypothyroidism) Gradual onset of constant, debilitating fatigue; feeling cold, slowed down. Skin may feel dry, hair brittle. Fingers and feet may feel swollen.	See GP as soon as possible for assessment and possible blood test.
Pregnancy Late, missed period. Nausea and sore breasts may occur several weeks before abdominal swelling is noticed.	Use a home pregnancy test; these are now as reliable as hospital tests.
Oedema (tissue swelling) Swelling first of feet, then legs and rest of body. Pressing a finger into the affected part for ten seconds will leave a visible dimple that takes minutes to clear. Many underlying causes including congestive heart failure.	See GP as soon as possible, urgently if short of breath or very ill.
Excess alcohol Signs of excess alcohol such as lifestyle factors (eg spending too long in the pub), red face and palms. Abdomen usually noticeably enlarged. Muscles may be wasted and thin.	Stop drinking. See GP as soon as possible for assessment; seek help from drugs and alcohol agency.

Weight loss, excessive

The concept of normal weight is defined by the Body Mass Index (see above). Any weight loss that is unexpected and rapid should be investigated, even if the person is not underweight.

OCCASIONAL CAUSES: drug, alcohol or laxative misuse; heart failure; chronic kidney and liver failure; undiagnosed diabetes mellitus; chronic inflammatory conditions (eg rheumatoid arthritis); gastro-intestinal disease (eg peptic ulcer, inflammatory bowel disease, coeliac disease, parasites).
RARE CAUSES: any chronic infection (especially tuberculosis); endocrine disorder; AIDS; malnutrition.

COMMON CAUSES	ACTION
Stress from life events Mild anxiety symptoms, such as tremor, fast heartbeat, nervous emotional state, associated with obvious life event (eg relationship breakup). Loss of appetite possible.	Consider ways to reduce life stress and increase relaxation. See GP if weight loss continues.
Depressive illness Tiredness that may vary with time of day; tearfulness; loss of confidence, concentration, pleasure, self-esteem. Poor sleep.	If present for two weeks or more, see GP as soon as possible. Should respond to treatment.
Eating disorders (anorexia nervosa, bulimia nervosa) **Anorexia**: inappropriate, unshakeable self-image of being overweight; extreme dieting, possibly self-induced vomiting. **Bulimia**: binge-eating alternates with starvation diet, self-induced vomiting common; disordered eating habits.	See GP as soon as possible: these are serious and need expert help. May respond to behavioural treatment; antidepressants can be very helpful.
Hyperthyroidism (overactive thyroid) Gradual, relentless weight loss; fast heartbeat with missed beats. Associated with feeling hot and dislike of warm environments; fine tremor of hands.	See GP as soon as possible for assessment.
Cancer Rapid weight loss, loss of appetite. Feeling very unwell.	See GP as soon as possible.

Breathlessness, chronic

Breathlessness is the sensation of having to breathe harder than expected for a given level of activity. For example, panting when just walking on level ground, or even having to breathe hard when at rest. It is said to be chronic when it occurs over a long period of time, months or years.

OCCASIONAL CAUSES: bronchiectasis (widening of bronchial air passages); recurrent pulmonary emboli (clots blocking lung arterioles); large hiatus hernia; lung cancer with collapse of part of a lung (lobar collapse); pleural effusion (fluid in lung lining). **RARE CAUSES:** pulmonary fibrosis; motor neurone disease; muscular dystrophy.

COMMON CAUSES	ACTION
Obesity Breathlessness occurs in people who are obviously obese. It may be worse when lying down.	Seek dietary advice and ensure clothes are not too tight.
Chronic obstructive pulmonary disease (COPD) Chronic cough and production of phlegm. Nearly always the result of smoking.	Stop smoking. See GP non-urgently for assessment, treatment and possible referral.
Anaemia Pale lips, tongue and insides of eyelids. Increasing fatigue may develop alongside the shortness of breath.	See GP as soon as possible for blood test to confirm the diagnosis and further assessment.
Congestive cardiac failure Always worse on lying down. Ankle swelling, with possible wheezy cough and phlegm.	See GP as soon as possible for assessment and treatment.
Asthma Wheezing and cough brought on by exertion or exposure to allergens such as cats, dogs or pollen.	See GP as soon as possible for assessment and treatment.

Breathlessness, sudden

This is the sudden inability to breathe, or a sudden sensation of not being able to breathe enough for a given level of activity. There is a sense of suffocation or 'hunger for air'. Sudden breathlessness is always a very distressing and frightening experience. Blueish lips (cyanosis) or confusion indicate a severe shortage of oxygen: dial 999 immediately.

OCCASIONAL CAUSES: pneumothorax (air leaking from lung); pulmonary embolism (clot); pleural effusion (fluid in lung lining); severe biochemical imbalance (diabetic ketoacidosis); collapse of part of a lung (lobar collapse) caused by a cancerous tumour. **RARE CAUSES:** hypovolaemic shock (lack of blood); obstruction of the windpipe by foreign body.

COMMON CAUSES	ACTION
Acute asthmatic attack Severe difficulty in breathing, with wheezing and drawing in of the skin between the ribs. Inability to speak indicates an extremely severe attack.	Use medication if appropriate. Call GP urgently, or dial 999 if it appears very severe.
Pneumonia Fever, coughing up dirty-looking phlegm, fast breathing rate. Tearing chest pain in deep breathing indicates inflammation of the lung membranes (pleurisy).	Call GP urgently. Continue coughing up of phlegm and keep sitting upright.
Inefficient heart pumping (acute left ventricular failure) Severe shortness of breath on exertion, made worse by lying down. May come on suddenly during the night while asleep; can be the first sign of a heart attack (myocardial infarction).	Sit up in a chair with feet down to relieve the burden on the heart; this could save your life. Dial 999.
Exacerbation of chronic obstructive pulmonary disease (COPD) Long-standing lung disease (such as emphysema); similar features to those of Pneumonia, above.	Call GP urgently.
Hyperventilation (rapid breathing) Overwhelming anxiety. Very fast breathing rate, often associated with 'pins and needles' in fingers, toes and around mouth. Spasm of hands and feet may occur.	Calm symptoms: breathe in and out of a paper bag held over mouth and nose. Call GP urgently for advice.

Chest pain, sudden

Chest pain can take many forms: it may be dull or sharp, aching or stabbing, constant or throbbing, in one place or all over the chest. It may also be referred, felt in another part of the body. For example, heart pain can be felt in the arms, neck and jaw.

OCCASIONAL CAUSES: lung membrane inflammation (pleurisy); peptic ulcer; gallstones; shingles; mastitis (inflammation of the breast).
RARE CAUSES: pulmonary infarct (clot in the lung); inflammation of the heart (eg pericarditis, myocarditis); fractured ribs; dissecting aortic aneurysm (tearing in a swelling of the aorta).

COMMON CAUSES	ACTION
Angina, heart attack (myocardial infarction) Severe, crushing central pain; may be felt in jaw, neck and arms. Nausea; breathlessness; sweaty skin; faintness. Angina is precipitated by exertion and settles with rest. A heart attack may occur at rest and does not settle with rest.	Dial 999 and take half a 300mg aspirin tablet, if not allergic or sensitive to it, to reduce the risk of blood clots (thrombosis).
Reflux oesophagitis (inflammation of the gullet) Anything from mild acid heartburn to symptoms similar to those of Angina, above. Usually acid regurgitation in throat when stooping, lying down and after meals.	If severe, dial 999: requires tests to distinguish it from heart pain. If mild, try OTC antacids or a milky drink.
Anxiety (Da Costa's syndrome) Pain often in one specific point in the chest; related to a stressful event or generally anxious personality.	See GP as soon as possible.
Pulled muscle Usually after physical activity; triggered by certain arm movements. Sore point in affected muscle.	Gentle activity to prevent stiffness. Take OTC anti-inflammatories, painkillers.
Inflammation of the rib cartilage (costochondritis) Often triggered by a general viral illness. Pain on deep breathing in a few points between ribs and breastbone, which are sore to touch.	Take OTC anti-inflammatories, painkillers.

Cough

A cough is a sudden, explosive release of air from the lungs through the mouth. The urge to cough is often a ticklish, irritating sensation, felt in the throat or windpipe. Coughs are often described as productive (with phlegm) or dry (without phlegm). Always see a GP for a cough continuing for six weeks or more. Smoking can be a contributory factor in all of the common causes listed.

OCCASIONAL CAUSES: lung tumour; inefficient heart pumping (left ventricular failure); side effect of ACE inhibitors (high blood pressure drugs); psychological factors.
RARE CAUSES: ear wax or foreign body in ear canal; inhaled foreign body; tuberculosis; cystic fibrosis; cancer of the larynx.

COMMON CAUSES	ACTION
Infection of the upper airways Often follows or accompanies a sore throat or cold. Green or yellow phlegm common in first few days.	Try OTC remedies, steam inhalations. Avoid smoky atmospheres. See GP if not improving after a week.
Chest infection Fever, hot and cold sweats, feeling very unwell; copious yellow, green or brown phlegm that may be bloodstained. In severe cases there may be shortness of breath.	See GP urgently for examination and antibiotic treatment.
Asthma Dry cough, possibly with wheeze, difficulty breathing and chest tightness. Asthma often triggered by emotion, exertion or exposure to allergens such as dogs, cats, pollen.	See GP as soon as possible for examination and treatment.
Nose area inflammations (rhinitis, chronic sinusitis) Stuffy nose with persistent catarrh dripping down back of throat. Sinusitis causes pain over and/or under eyes, and the pain throbs on walking and stooping.	Try OTC remedies. Avoid smoke. See GP if not improving after a week.
Inflammation of the gullet (oesophageal reflux) Acid regurgitation in throat, often on stooping or lying down. Heartburn, often made worse by hot drinks and spicy foods.	Try OTC antacids; avoid trigger foods. See GP if problem continues.

Coughing up blood

Blood can be coughed up from the windpipe or lungs, either on its own or mixed with phlegm. Most of the serious causes listed here are rare; most commonly the blood is from the nose or mouth or caused by a chest infection. But if breathing is difficult phone a GP for urgent advice or dial 999.

OCCASIONAL CAUSES:
mitral stenosis (a narrowing of the heart valve opening); bronchiectasis (widening of air passages); polyarteritis nodosa (an inflammation of the artery walls); tuberculosis; tumour of larynx or trachea.
RARE CAUSES: injury-related bruising of the brain (contusion).

COMMON CAUSES	ACTION
Chest infection You will be feeling unwell, have a fever and be coughing up copious yellow, green or brown phlegm. Shortness of breath indicates a severe infection.	Drink plenty of non-alcoholic fluids. See GP urgently or ask for home visit if necessary.
Blood clot on the lung (pulmonary embolism) Sudden shortness of breath and chest pain on deep breathing. May be preceded by calf pain, signifying deep vein thrombosis.	See GP urgently; if breathing is difficult dial 999.
Lung cancer Generally feeling unwell, usually preceded by weight loss, shortness of breath. Rare in non-smokers.	See GP as soon as possible for assessment.
Fluid in the lung (pulmonary oedema) May occur without warning, often while sleeping. Phlegm is pink and frothy. Swollen ankles; severe shortness of breath, made worse by lying down.	Sit in chair with feet down. Dial 999.
Prolonged coughing Coughing is painful. Often linked with a viral infection (eg a cold), but can occur with any cause of cough (see page 23).	Take frequent sips of cold drinks. Try steam inhalations and humidification.

Palpitations

Palpitations are abnormal-feeling heartbeats, such as fast or irregular ones. They are uncomfortable and often feel like a fluttering in the chest or lower neck. An occasional missed beat (ectopic beat) is normal. Palpitations are more likely to represent a medical problem in people aged over 60 than in younger people.

OCCASIONAL CAUSES:
heart disorders (eg mitral valve disease, cardiomyopathy); electrolyte abnormality (a blood disorder); alcohol abuse; anaemia.
RARE CAUSES: tumour in the chest cavity (a mediastinal tumour); pulmonary embolism (a blood clot in the lung); inflammation of the heart muscle (myocarditis).

COMMON CAUSES	ACTION
Anxiety Fast, racing heartbeat or runs of missed beats lasting seconds or minutes. Nervous emotional state; life stresses likely. Sweaty skin, shaky hands; breathlessness and pins and needles common.	Consider ways to reduce life stress. See GP as soon as possible for confirmation and help (see also page 19).
Missed beats Occasional and infrequent missed beats in an otherwise healthy person. May occur several times a day, but there should not be more than six in one minute.	No action necessary. If there are consistently more than six missed beats per minute, see GP non-urgently.
Overactive thyroid (thyrotoxicosis) Consistently fast heartbeat with missed beats. Gradual, relentless weight loss; feeling hot with dislike of warm environments. Fine tremor of hands.	See GP as soon as possible for assessment.
Heart attack (myocardial infarction) Usually sudden onset of fast and/or irregular heartbeat; with crushing central chest pain that may travel to arms, neck and jaw. Shortness of breath, faintness and nausea.	Dial 999 for ambulance. Take half a 300mg aspirin tablet if not allergic, asthmatic or with stomach problems.
Ischaemic heart disease (blood vessel blockage) Runs of fast and/or irregular heartbeats, brought on by exertion. Often associated with angina (see page 23).	See GP as soon as possible, urgently if this is a new problem and if faint and/or short of breath.

Hair loss

Hair loss may affect just one part of the scalp, appear in patches, or occur in a symmetrical pattern as in male baldness. It is usually painless, unless it is caused by a painful inflammation. Hair loss can affect the whole body.

OCCASIONAL CAUSES:
bacterial folliculitis (inflammation of the hair follicles); telogen effluvium (a form of alopecia, involving sudden hair loss but regrowth after a time); endocrine disorders (eg myxoedema, hypopituitarism and hypoparathyroidism); lupus erythematosus (an inflammatory disease); side effect of chemotherapy.
RARE CAUSES: secondary syphilis; trichotillomania (ingrained habit of rubbing, fiddling with or pulling hair out); alopecia totalis (an autoimmune condition).

COMMON CAUSES

COMMON CAUSES	ACTION
Male pattern baldness (androgenic alopecia) The scalp is normal. Patchy hair loss works backwards from the forehead, and is more pronounced above the temples. Also thinning crown. 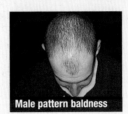 Male pattern baldness	There is no reliably proven treatment that works for everyone but two marketed 'cures' appear to slow hair loss for some of their users – minoxidil (Regaine) and finasteride (Propecia).
Seborrhoeic dermatitis (fungal infection) Scaly crusts on scalp, often weeping clear fluid. There may be a similar scaly rash on parts of the body.	Control symptoms with OTC antifungal selenium-containing shampoos.
Alopecia areata (bald patches) Patchy hair thinning on a normal scalp. The hairs are tapered, thin towards the ends, like exclamation marks (can be seen under a magnifying glass). 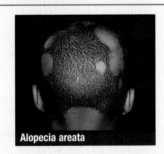 Alopecia areata	See GP non-urgently for confirmation. Rarely there is an association with uncommon autoimmune diseases.
Allergic dermatitis Patchy hair thinning with a reddened inflamed scalp. There may be similar rashes on the body. Follows use of allergens such as scalp lotion, shampoo.	Avoid allergen if possible. Steroid creams will settle this: see GP non-urgently for advice.
Tinea capitis (fungal infection) Patchy hair thinning, with scaly weeping around areas of scalp. There may be similar ring-shaped areas of skin on the body. 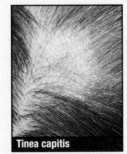 Tinea capitis	Use OTC antifungal creams. If you have a cat or dog, get it checked by a vet as it may carry the fungus.

Itching

In general, itching is made worse by anything that increases the blood supply to the skin, including alcohol and heat. Calamine lotion, OTC antihistamine tablets or hydrocortisone cream can offer relief. If itching persists for more than a few days, see a GP.

OCCASIONAL CAUSES: ingested allergens such as food (eg strawberries and shellfish) and drugs; jaundice; iron-deficiency anaemia; endocrine disorders (eg diabetes mellitus, hypothyroidism, hyperthyroidism); kidney failure.
RARE CAUSES: psychological factors; diseases of white blood cells (eg leukaemia); itching of unknown cause.

COMMON CAUSES	ACTION
Contact dermatitis Itchy, inflamed and sometimes weeping skin in one area, where contact with the allergen has been made. 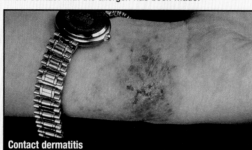 Contact dermatitis	Avoid allergen. Nickel jewellery or jeans studs are common allergens.
Scabies and other skin infestations Furiously itchy rash, which often spreads from the hands and is worse at night. 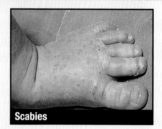 Scabies	Try OTC antiscabies lotion; itching may last up to ten days after end of treatment. Contagious by direct contact only.
Atopic eczema (a skin disease) Itchy, flaky, inflamed and sometimes weeping skin, often in the bends of the arms and legs. 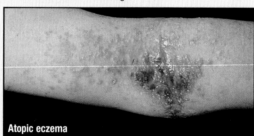 Atopic eczema	Try OTC hydrocortisone cream. See GP if not settling within a week. May need antibiotic cream.
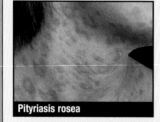 Pityriasis rosea **Pityriasis rosea (skin rash)** Raised, reddened spots 5mm–2cm (¼–¾in) long. Oval patches in characteristic 'Christmas tree' pattern, with long axes pointing the same way. Often starts with one large patch. Takes six weeks to develop and fade.	Try OTC treatments to help symptoms; there is no cure. It is probably caused by a virus, and always goes away on its own.
Psoriasis Raised, reddened patches from 5mm to many centimetres (¼–2in) in size. Silvery scaling may be seen when scratched. 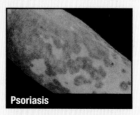 Psoriasis	See GP as soon as possible. There are no effective home treatments.

Blisters

Blisters are categorized into two types according to their size: vesicles are up to 5mm (¼in) in diameter and bullae are more than 5mm (¼in) in diameter. They may be filled with a clear, straw-coloured fluid (lymph) or blood. Blisters may be painless with no unusual sensations or they may be associated with feelings of itching, pain or burning. For blisters filled with pus, see Pus spots, page 32.

OCCASIONAL CAUSES: autoimmune skin disorders (eg pemphigus, pemphigoid); scabies (tiny blisters); dermatitis herpetiformis (a condition that resembles herpes virus infection); bullous impetigo (a skin infection); drug eruption; erythema multiforme (spots are symmetrical with a central blister, like targets).
RARE CAUSES: porphyria (a metabolic disorder); epidermolysis bullosa (a genetic disorder); allergic vasculitis (inflammation of the blood vessels).

COMMON CAUSES

Injury
Injury usually visible and with obvious cause such as friction, heat, chemical burns or insect bites. Blisters usually more than 5mm (¼in) in diameter.

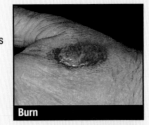
Burn

Cold sore (herpes simplex)
Crop of blisters in one area, usually on or around mouth and less than 5mm (¼in) in diameter. Blisters are preceded by skin tingling and pain.

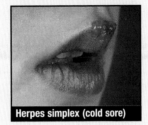
Herpes simplex (cold sore)

Shingles (herpes zoster)
Blisters are usually less than 5mm (¼in) in diameter. Always on one side of the body, spreading out in a band around the trunk or down a limb. Pain not helped by OTC painkillers.

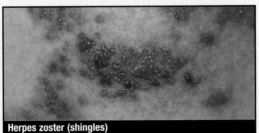
Herpes zoster (shingles)

Childhood viruses
Chickenpox or hand, foot and mouth disease may be the cause. Sufferer may feel mildly ill, as with a cold, before rash appears. Neck glands may be enlarged.

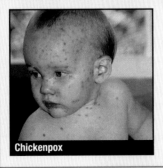
Chickenpox

Eczema
Blisters are often more than 5mm (¼in) in diameter, and may be painful. Commonly on hands, palms or soles of feet.

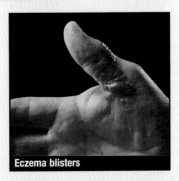
Eczema blisters

ACTION

Do not burst blister; cover with dry plaster. See GP urgently if redness is spreading out from blister and pain increases, since infection is possible.

Apply OTC antiviral cream as soon as possible. See GP urgently if rash spreads beyond original crop.

See GP urgently; antiviral treatment may be needed. It is contagious: avoid contact with adults who have not had chickenpox, especially pregnant women, until the last blister has burst and scabbed over.

See GP as soon as possible for confirmation. Viral illnesses are contagious: see recommendations for Shingles, above.

See GP as soon as possible, urgently if the skin is very painful – this is unusual and may indicate that the skin is infected or cracked.

Symptom sorter

Bruising

Bruising is reddish-purple skin discoloration that does not whiten under pressure. The medical name is purpura.

OCCASIONAL CAUSES: painful bruising syndrome; connective tissue disorders (eg lupus erythematosis); vasculitis (inflammation of blood vessel walls); platelet (blood) defects. RARE CAUSES: bone marrow damage (caused by cytotoxic drugs, leukaemia or cancer); inherited blood-clotting disorders (eg haemophilia); infections (eg meningococcal septicaemia); deficiency of vitamin C or K.

COMMON CAUSES

ACTION

Injury
Bruises can be any size, and are usually tender to the touch. The original injury is often minor.

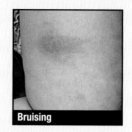
Bruising

No treatment needed, but cold compresses reduce swelling and arnica cream may help to speed up recovery. If repeated bruising appears on areas not subjected to everyday knocks, see a GP as soon as possible.

Senile purpura (age-related bruising)
Bruises often appears repeatedly, are widespread and without obvious cause. This is caused by fragile blood vessels in ageing skin.

See GP as soon as possible if there is unexplained bleeding of any sort as well; otherwise no action needed.

Liver disease (especially alcoholic cirrhosis)
Widespread bruises of all sizes repeatedly appear. There may be other signs of liver disease or alcohol excess.

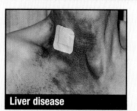
Liver disease

See GP urgently: there may be a blood-clotting problem.

Coughing or vomiting
Tiny bruises appear on the face immediately after a violent coughing fit or vomiting, which increases pressure in major blood vessels. Also seen inside lips and eyelids.

No action needed: it looks alarming but is of no importance in itself.

Drug reactions
Widespread tiny bruises appear suddenly. They are not painful, but you may feel unwell from some other side effect of the drug (eg steroids, aspirin, warfarin, quinine, thiazides).

See GP as soon as possible; urgently if you are taking warfarin.

Special care: meningitis

Meningitis is an infection of the membranes surrounding the brain and spinal cord (the meninges). Meningitis is very rare, but all parents and carers should know how to recognize it.

The symptoms of meningitis are:
- feeling very unwell, with a fever;
- severe, throbbing headache;
- feeling sick, or vomiting;
- intense dislike of bright light (photophobia), including indoor lighting;
- stiff (not just sore) neck; difficult to turn head;
- floppiness and sleepiness in babies and young children. Older children may be unusually drowsy.

A purplish rash that doesn't fade when pressure is put on the skin is a late and serious sign of the illness. The glass test (see below) can help you to tell whether or not a rash is non-blanching.

All these symptoms can be caused by common illnesses, including migraine and non-serious virus infections. If in doubt phone your GP for advice.

The glass test
Take an ordinary clear glass or plastic tumbler. Place it on the skin next to the spots. Roll it onto the spots, applying firm pressure. Note that the normal skin under the glass goes white as the blood is pushed out of the tiny surface blood vessels.

Meningitis may be indicated if a spot does not fade when the glass is rolled onto it. Call an ambulance if this is the case in an ill child.

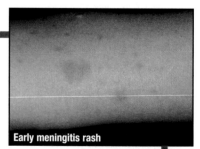
Early meningitis rash

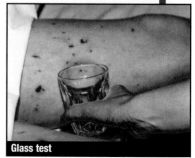
Glass test

Flat spots

Flat spots are any abnormally coloured, flat areas of skin; the medical term is macules. They vary in colour from red, white to brown, black and grey. Purple or dark red bruises are called purpura (see page 28). Some red flat spots share causes with erythema (see Red rash, page 33).

OCCASIONAL CAUSES: measles; German measles (rubella); post-inflammatory pigmentation; café-au-lait spots (creamy brown spots); Mongolian spots (brown, slate-grey spots); skin sensitivity to light (photosensitivity) as a reaction to certain chemicals (eg oil of bergamot, used in perfume); depigmentation (white spots). **RARE CAUSES:** infections; Albright's syndrome; neurofibromatosis (a nervous system disorder – often heralded by five or more large, coffee-coloured patches); pathological freckles (freckles caused by sun damage; don't fade in winter and may indicate early skin cancer).

COMMON CAUSES	ACTION
Allergy or drug reaction Itchy, red, burning spots, often more than 5mm (¼in) in diameter.	See GP urgently if you suspect a drug reaction. If not, try OTC antihistamines.
Flat mole (junctional naevus) Brown spots, often with variable depth of colour; small ones look like freckles. Can be several centimetres (1–2in) in diameter. 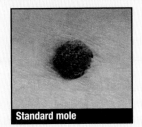 Standard mole	No action needed. If it is regularly subjected to damage, changes in size or colour, or becomes lumpy, see GP as soon as possible; this may indicate melanoma.
Non-specific viral rash Red and frequently large area of skin that is painless and does not itch.	No treatment needed unless illness itself requires medical advice.
Sun-induced freckles Crops of tiny, flat, brown spots, often appearing on face and arms but also found elsewhere. Usually seen in summer. 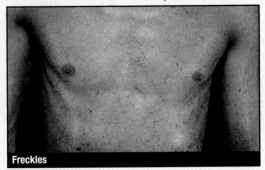 Freckles	No action needed.
Chloasma (reaction to sunlight) Mask-like, symmetrical brown area on front of the face. Affects women only, especially those who are pregnant or who take a combined oral contraceptive pill. 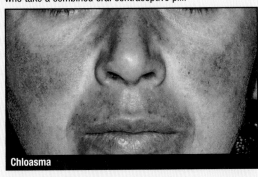 Chloasma	No action needed if you are pregnant; if on contraceptive pill, see GP as soon as possible.

Symptom sorter

Lumps (nodules)

Lumps of more than 5mm (¼in) in diameter, located within or just beneath the skin, are called nodules. Smaller lumps are called papules (see page 31). Nodules are usually visible to the naked eye, and are usually painless and not itchy, although this depends on the cause. They feel like a firm or hard lump in the skin.

COMMON CAUSES | ACTION

Sebaceous cyst (blocked grease gland in skin)
Firm or hard lump fixed to the skin, with a central hole or dimple (punctum).

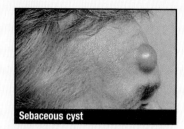
Sebaceous cyst

No treatment needed as a sebaceous cyst is harmless, unless causing other problems. See GP non-urgently. Do not squeeze, as it may become inflamed.

Rodent ulcer (basal cell cancer)
Reddish-brown lump with rolled-up, pearly edge, often with tiny blood vessels in it. Central area often ulcerates. It is common in sun-exposed areas (such as the forehead, nose, cheeks, tips of ears and forearms).

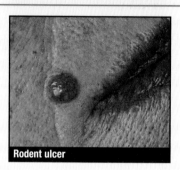
Rodent ulcer

See GP as soon as possible; the lump can be removed by simple surgery under local anaesthetic. It almost never spreads beyond the area immediately around it.

Viral wart
Usually solitary, hard and painless lump on skin surface, but may occur in crops. Common on fingers. On feet viral warts are known as verrucas, and may become painful from the pressure of walking.

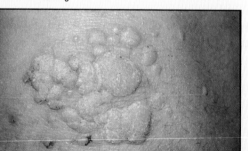
Viral warts

Try OTC remedies. See GP non-urgently if these fail.

OCCASIONAL CAUSES:
squamous cell carcinoma (a type of skin cancer); kerato-acanthoma (a harmless, rapidly growing but self-curing skin lump); benign tumour (histiocytoma); gout; lumps on the small joints of fingers, seen in rheumatoid arthritis and osteoarthritis (rheumatoid nodules and Heberden's nodes); pyogenic granuloma (a chronic inflammatory lump that bleeds readily).
RARE CAUSES: cancers (eg skin and secondary, lymphoma); vasculitis (inflammation of the blood vessels); uncommon infections (eg leprosy).

Lipoma (benign tumour)
Soft, smooth, mobile round lump under the skin, which can reach 10cm (4in) in diameter or more.

See GP non-urgently.

Lumps (papules)

Solid, marked skin lumps with a definite circumference, up to 5mm (¼in) in diameter, are called papules. Larger lumps are known as nodules (see opposite). Papules may be painful or painless, depending on the cause, and may develop into something else.

OCCASIONAL CAUSES: xanthelasma (fat deposits around eyelids); molluscum contagiosum (a viral problem); guttate psoriasis (scaly skin lumps); skin diseases (eg lichen planus); insect bites.

RARE CAUSES: cancers (eg melanoma, early basal cell carcinoma, Kaposi's sarcoma); acanthosis nigricans (skin thickening associated with stomach cancer); naevoxantho-endothelioma (rounded yellow, firm lumps that appear within a few weeks of birth and disappear within 1–3 years); pseudoxanthoma elasticum (an inherited condition that affects the neck and armpits especially); tuberous sclerosis (cysts and lumps that become calcified and affect many different organs).

COMMON CAUSES

Blocked sweat gland ducts (milia)
Painless crops of solid white spots, often on eyelids or cheeks.

Acne (acne vulgaris)
Firm, painful lumps that go on to enlarge, develop a yellow head with surrounding inflammation, then burst. May scar on healing.

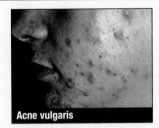
Acne vulgaris

Viral wart
Usually solitary, hard, painless lump on skin surface, but may occur in crops. Common on fingers. On feet they are called verrucas, and may become painful from pressure of walking.

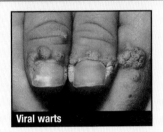
Viral warts

Xanthoma (fat deposits in the skin)
Multiple reddish brown or yellow-whitish lumps, often found around the eyes.

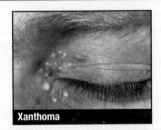
Xanthoma

Campbell de Morgan spot (cherry spots or angioma)
Bright red round spots, usually on the trunk. They are more common with increasing age.

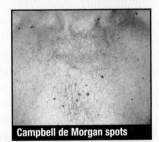
Campbell de Morgan spots

Skin tag (acrochordon)
Finger-like projection of skin. Common in armpits and on neck, and more common with increasing age.

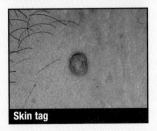
Skin tag

ACTION

Only treatment is good hygiene. Do not squeeze spots; this causes infection.

Practise good hygiene. Contrary to popular belief, a healthier diet will not clear up acne. See GP non-urgently if OTC remedies fail.

Try OTC remedies. See GP non-urgently if these fail.

See GP non-urgently: xanthoma may indicate high blood cholesterol level.

Completely harmless. Requires no medical treatment.

No treatment needed but may become large and uncomfortable. See GP non-urgently if a skin tag is a problem.

Symptom sorter

Pus spots

Pus spots (pustules) are raised skin lumps that are less than 5mm (¼in) in diameter and filled with pus. They are usually, but not always, caused by infection and can occur anywhere on the body. Avoid squeezing a pus spot, as this can spread infection into surrounding tissues. On and around the nose can be dangerous, as a link exists between the veins here and the large veins around the brain. Although they are very rare, cases of brain infection have been caused this way.

OCCASIONAL CAUSES: inflammation of the sweat gland in the armpits and groin (hidradenitis suppurativa); candidiasis; Staphylococcal (bacterial) infections (eg barber's rash/sycosis barbae); pustular psoriasis; dermatitis herpetiformis (inflamed and infected hair follicles).
RARE CAUSES: jacuzzi folliculitis (inflammation of the hair follicles caused by bacteria in jacuzzis).

COMMON CAUSES

Boil and carbuncle
A boil is a solitary pus spot. A carbuncle has several heads.

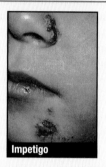
Boil

Impetigo and folliculitis (infections)
Impetigo: crops of golden-yellow pus spots, often on the hands or around the mouth. Common in children.
Folliculitis: often affects regularly shaved areas of body; crops of pustules on hair follicles.

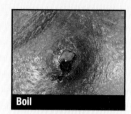
Impetigo

Cold sore (herpes simplex)
Skin tingling and pain precedes crop of blisters, usually less than 5mm (¼in) diameter, in one place.

Acne (acne vulgaris)
Firm, painful lumps which go on to enlarge, develop a yellow head with surrounding inflammation, then burst. May scar on healing.

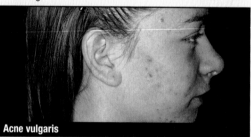
Acne vulgaris

Acne rosacea
Red rash on cheeks, bridge of nose and forehead in 'butterfly' distribution. Pus spots may or may not be present.

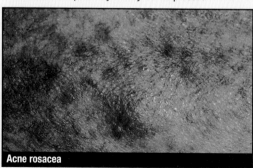
Acne rosacea

ACTION

Cover with dry, non-waterproof dressing. See GP as soon as possible for a carbuncle, or for a boil that has not burst on its own after five days.

Impetigo is highly infectious, so practise good hygiene. See GP urgently to halt infection.

Apply OTC antiviral cream as soon as possible. See GP urgently if rash spreads beyond original crop.

Practise good hygiene. Contrary to popular belief, diet makes no difference. Try OTC remedies; see GP non-urgently if these fail.

See GP as soon as possible.

Red rash

Red rashes are either flushing (see page 63), which disappears in a few minutes, or erythema, which lasts for hours or days. Eyrthema is caused by relaxation of blood vessels in the skin, which increases the circulation of blood to the skin. Unlike bruising (see page 28), the affected area whitens under pressure. It may be sore, painful or itchy depending on the cause.

OCCASIONAL CAUSES: viral rashes; palmar erythema (red palms); reaction to cold (especially in children); recurrent drug reaction; erythema multiforme (target-like spots) – a reaction to infections, drugs or for no known reason.
RARE CAUSES: HIV; erythema nodosum (painful lumps on the shin); prolonged exposure to heat (erythema ab igne); Lyme disease (from deer tics).

COMMON CAUSES	ACTION
Cellulitis (skin infection) An area of skin anywhere on the body is red, hot and painful to the touch. You feel unwell, with possible fever.	See GP urgently.
Gout Swollen joint, commonly big toe 'knuckle', top of foot or knee, is extremely painful to touch or move. Skin around the joint is red and hot. In severe cases there may be fever. 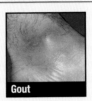 Gout	See GP urgently.
Burns The skin is very painful to touch and blistering may be present. Heat, contact with a chemical or sunburn may be the cause.	Keep skin cool and dry. Do not use ointments. If burn is large or skin is peeling, go to casualty.
Toxic erythema The skin is not usually painful. Fever and blistering possible. You feel generally unwell. Underlying cause may be a viral infection or drug reaction.	Try OTC antihistamine tablets if itchy. See GP urgently to check if drug reaction, or if very ill with viral infection.
Acne rosacea Rash on cheeks, bridge of nose and forehead in 'butterfly' distribution. Pus spots may be present.	See GP as soon as possible.

Scaly rash and plaque

A scaly rash is a dry, flaky area of skin, nearly always itchy. When it is thickened and raised it is called a plaque. Very serious causes are rare, and most common causes respond well to treatment. Avoid scratching as this will intensify the itching and cause it to spread or become infected. Try OTC antihistamines, hydrocortisone cream or calamine lotion.

OCCASIONAL CAUSES: lichen planus (itchy; usually scaly only on legs); precancerous sun-induced damage (solar keratosis); discoid (disc-shaped) eczema; pityriasis versicolor (skin depigmentation caused by yeast overgrowth); guttate psoriasis (causing scaly lumps).
RARE CAUSES: chronic dermatitis (parapsoriasis).

COMMON CAUSES	ACTION
Psoriasis (chronic skin disease) Raised reddened patches 5mm to many centimetres (¼in or more) in size. Silvery scaling may be seen when scratched.	See GP as soon as possible. There are no effective home treatments.
Atopic eczema and contact dermatitis Itchy, flaky, inflamed and sometimes weeping skin. In atopic eczema it often occurs in the bends of the arms and legs; contact dermatitis often appears on hands.	Try OTC hydrocortisone cream. See GP if not settling within a week. May need antibiotic cream.
Tinea/ringworm (fungal infection) In tinea corporis (ringworm) there is a red ring on the body that slowly expands, leaving a dry, scaly central area. In tinea cruris, there is a red, moist, itchy area in the groin.	Try OTC antifungal cream. See GP if this fails.
Seborrhoeic dermatitis (fungal infection) Scaly crusts on scalp, often weeping clear fluid. There may be a similar scaly rash on other parts of the body.	Control symptoms with OTC antifungal selenium-containing shampoos.
Pityriasis rosea (skin disorder) Patterns of raised, reddened oval spots 5mm–2cm (¼–¾in) long, with lengths of the ovals pointing the same way. Often starts with one large patch, and mostly affects trunk and tops of the arms and legs. Takes six weeks to develop and fade.	Try OTC treatments to help symptoms. There is no known cure but the rash, which is probably caused by a virus, always goes away on its own.

Arm pain

Arm pain can be any sort of pain: dull or sharp, constant or throbbing, aching or shooting, mild or severe, depending on the cause. The same condition, even if serious, can cause a variety of types of pain in different people.

OCCASIONAL CAUSES: subacromial bursitis (a form of tissue inflammation); neuritis (nerve inflammation in eg the neck, including post-shingles pain); cervical and thoracic disc prolapse; frozen shoulder.
RARE CAUSES: cancer of the spinal cord and brachial plexus (a network of major nerves); multiple sclerosis.

COMMON CAUSES	ACTION
Tennis elbow (lateral epicondylitis) Pain on bony lump on outer elbow going down back of arm to hand. Gripping and picking things up painful.	Try tennis player's sport support. Rest hand. See GP non-urgently.
Carpal tunnel syndrome (compressed nerve in wrist) Weak grip, tingling in hand especially at night or after using hand for manual task.	Rest hand, and elevate affected arm at night. See GP non-urgently.
Arthritis of the neck (cervical spondylosis) Pain often comes from neck; there may be a grating sensation in the neck.	Try OTC anti-inflammatories or painkillers. See GP non-urgently.
De Quervain's tenosynovitis (tendon inflammation) Pain just above wrist starts after prolonged repetitive actions such as using a screwdriver. Often affects use of thumb.	Prompt treatment with rest and anti-inflammatories important. See GP as soon as possible.
Angina (insufficient oxygen in heart blood) Usually associated with crushing chest pain, cold sweat and shortness of breath. Brought on by physical exertion, cold environment and sometimes large meals.	If severe, with these associations, and lasts more than 15 minutes, call GP urgently or dial 999 for ambulance. If intermittent, see GP as soon as possible.

Foot pain

Foot pain can have any character: it may be dull or sharp, constant or throbbing, aching or shooting, mild or severe, depending on the cause. If there is fever and a feeling of being unwell, infection is likely; see a GP urgently for treatment and to rule out the rare but serious bone infection osteomyelitis.

OCCASIONAL CAUSES: chilblains; foot bone damage; arthritis (osteo and rheumatoid); Achilles tendonitis/bursitis (inflammations); oedema (fluid accumulation).
RARE CAUSES: march fracture (a break in one of the long metatarsal bones, caused by jarring); bone infections (eg septic arthritis, osteomyelitis); blockage of the blood vessel (ischaemia).

COMMON CAUSES	ACTION
Gout Sudden onset of pain. The joint, commonly the 'knuckle' of the big toe, is red, hot, and painful to touch or move.	See GP urgently for treatment and blood test to confirm.
Inflamed sole ligaments (plantar fasciitis) Sensation of walking on a pebble in the sole of the foot. Often comes on after an unusual amount of walking.	Try OTC anti-inflammatories and a heel-raise wedge in shoe. If unsuccessful after a month, see GP non-urgently.
Bunion and displacement of big toe (hallux valgus) Tender, bony lump on side of knuckle joint of big toe, which is pointing outwards. Bunion	See chiropodist for corrective pads. If unsuccessful and severe, see GP for possible orthopaedic referral/surgery.
Ingrowing toenail, infected Edge of big toe nail is buried in nail fold, which is red, very painful and may leak pus. Ingrowing toenail	See GP urgently for antibiotics. When infection is cured, see chiropodist for corrective treatment; if unsuccessful, see GP for minor surgery.
Verruca (foot wart) Gradual onset of pain. Painful flat, warty lump on sole of foot.	Try OTC treatments. See chiropodist to have it filed down regularly.

Calf pain

This is pain in the back of the leg, between the knee and ankle. It may be felt just in the skin or, more deeply, in the muscle of the calf. The type of pain varies and does not usually represent a serious condition.

OCCASIONAL CAUSES: referred pain from back or knee; alcoholic or diabetic neuropathy (nerve disease); hypocalcaemic cramps (painful spasms as a result of abnormally low blood calcium levels); ruptured Baker's cyst (cysts caused by fluid build-up behind knee in disorders such as rheumatoid arthritis); superficial thrombophlebitis (inflammation of the vein wall); deep vein thrombosis (blood clot).
RARE CAUSES: motor neurone disease; multiple sclerosis; muscle tension.

COMMON CAUSES	ACTION
Cramp May be brought on by exercise. The calf contracts violently and immediately becomes hard and painful. In elderly people, cramp is often worse at night.	Pull toes towards knee. See GP non-urgently if recurrent: possible blood mineral imbalance/circulatory problem.
Muscle stiffness Both calves sore the day after unaccustomed exercise. Pain reduces once the muscle is used again.	Gradually build up amount of exercise. Keep using legs and pain will settle.
Cellulitis (skin infection) Spreading area of hot, red, swollen skin. May follow a trivial wound or insect bite. Fever and feeling unwell possible.	See GP urgently: requires antibiotic treatment.
Peripheral vascular disease A blood circulation disorder (also called intermittent claudication), this causes cramp in one or both calves after walking. It disappears with rest and recurs after walking the same distance. Sufferers may have noticed cold feet or legs for some time before this starts happening.	See GP as soon as possible for further investigation. If no contra-indications, take half a 300mg aspirin daily to reduce risk of clot. If you smoke, stop.
Muscle injury (for instance, strain) Pain immediately after an injury. May progress to substantial swelling, redness of the calf and disability.	Apply cold compress straightaway to reduce swelling. To prevent disability, important to exercise muscle gently.

Joint pain, multiple

Pain in several joints at once can signify a general infection or disease (more likely in children and young adults), or a widespread inflammatory illness (more likely in people aged 40–60). Osteoarthritis (more common with increasing age) may affect several joints, or just one (see also page 36).

OCCASIONAL CAUSES: Reiter's syndrome (an inflammatory disorder); Paget's disease (of the bone); ankylosing spondylitis (an inflammatory disorder); vascular disease (eg giant-cell arteritis, polyarteritis nodosa); malignant tumours (usually secondary); corticosteroid drugs.
RARE CAUSES: unusual systemic infections that affect the whole body; decompression sickness (the bends).

COMMON CAUSES	ACTION
Rheumatoid arthritis Most common in women aged 20–40. Small joints of the hand, the wrists and ankles usually affected; nearly always affects both sides of body. Possibly generally unwell, with fever.	If the condition has not previously been diagnosed, see GP urgently for treatment and investigation.
Psoriatic joint disorder (arthropathy) Skin psoriasis has usually been present for a time already. Can affect any joint.	See GP as soon as possible; if no contra-indication, take OTC anti-inflammatories.
Viral polyarthritis More common before adulthood. Sudden feeling of being unwell, with a fever, often a few days after the start of a viral illness. Possible rash. Rheumatic fever is rare but has similar symptoms.	Rest and take OTC painkillers or anti-inflammatories; if not better after five days, contact GP for advice.
Systemic inflammatory diseases Usually a sign of some other illness already present, such as bowel problems, skin blisters or rash. Affects any age group. Does not usually improve on its own.	See GP as soon as possible for assessment and treatment.
Osteoarthritis, multiple Morning stiffness and night pain common. Pain improves with activity. Increasingly likely from age 50.	Try OTC anti-inflammatories or painkillers. See GP non-urgently.

Joint pain, single, sudden

A single joint may be painful in an otherwise well person, or it may occur with a pre-existing joint disease. The pain may be dull or sharp, constant or throbbing, aching or shooting, mild or severe, depending on the cause. The most common cause of sudden single joint pain is injury, and the joint most commonly affected is the knee.

OCCASIONAL CAUSES: fracture; inflammation of the kneecap (chondromalacia patellae); anterior (front) knee pain syndromes (eg patellar tendinitis); blood in the joint (haemarthrosis) causing it to swell, usually as a result of severe injury.
RARE CAUSES: tropical infections; malignant tumours (usually secondary).

COMMON CAUSES	ACTION
Flare-up of osteoarthritis Morning stiffness, swelling, night pain and improvement with activity. Usually a long history of previous problems with the same joint.	Try OTC anti-inflammatories or painkillers; see GP as soon as possible if not better within a week.
Torn ligament Similar to traumatic synovitis (see below), but it is almost impossible to use the joint.	Pain usually requires GP treatment, but worth trying cold compress, OTC anti-inflammatories or painkillers first.
Septic arthritis Severely painful, hot, red, swollen joint that can barely be moved or touched. Fever and general feeling of illness.	See GP urgently or ask for home visit: this emergency needs hospitalization.
Gout Very similar to septic arthritis (see above), but no fever or general feeling of illness. 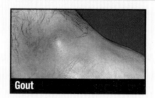 Gout	See GP urgently for diagnosis (blood test) and treatment.
Traumatic synovitis (inflammation) The joint is hot, red and swollen. There is no fever. The inflammation is caused by an injury, which is usually remembered.	Apply cold compress, try OTC painkillers or anti-inflammatories. See GP if not better within a week.

Limping in a child

A limp is an uneven gait. The vast majority of causes in children are not serious and will settle down in time; if it persists beyond a day or two without obvious cause, see a GP, especially if the limping child has a fever.

OCCASIONAL CAUSES: Perthes' disease (hip joint disease, usually in young boys); rheumatic fever; septic arthritis; deviation of the backbone (idiopathic scoliosis); congenital dislocation of the hip.
RARE CAUSES: bone inflammation (acute osteomyelitis); juvenile rheumatoid arthritis.

COMMON CAUSES	ACTION
Injury, including foreign body in foot There may or may not be obvious signs of injury.	Look at soles of feet for splinters and other objects. If injury obvious, see GP urgently, or go to casualty.
Irritable hip (transient synovitis) Child usually well; problem may start suddenly. The pain may be felt in the knee (referred pain).	See GP as soon as possible.
Acute viral infection, with joint pain Feeling unwell, following a viral infection (such as a cold or sore throat); fever common.	See GP urgently: can mimic rarer, more serious conditions.
Chronic juvenile arthritis Markedly stiff first thing in the morning. Fever possible and several joints likely to be affected.	See GP urgently: can mimic rarer, more serious conditions.
Slipped femoral epiphysis (end of thigh bone) Limp starts suddenly. Most common in boys who are overweight and aged over ten years old.	See GP urgently for assessment.

Nails, abnormal

Many diseases can alter the appearance of the nails, and doctors often start a general examination by looking at the nails. A chiropodist is often the best person to examine an abnormal toenail.

OCCASIONAL CAUSES: horizontal ridging may appear 6–8 weeks after severe illness because of interference with growth; longitudinal ridging (often no known cause); fungal infection of the nail fold (chronic paronychia); dermatitis; clubbing (shape change associated with lung cancer, chronic lung infection, cyanotic heart disease); autoimmune diseases (eg alopecia areata); spoon nails (associated with iron-deficiency anaemia).
RARE CAUSES: chronic cardiac failure; liver disease; lung tuberculosis; diabetes; rheumatoid arthritis; some cancers; poor circulation.

COMMON CAUSES	ACTION
Injury to nail bed Horizontal ridge on single nail appearing six to eight weeks after an injury such as a hammer blow.	No action needed.
Psoriasis Thickened white nail. Usually associated with a red scaly rash on the body.	Non-urgent GP appointment. Psoriasis needs treatment.
Onychomycosis (fungal infection) Thickened, white and crumbly nail. Can look indistinguishable from psoriasis. 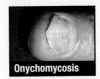 Onychomycosis	Non-urgent GP appointment for a lab test on the nail and treatment if positive.
Injury due to biting, hangnail Nails have ragged edges. The adjoining skin is often softened and sore.	Stop biting the nails. Bitter nail paints may help.
Onychogryphosis (thickening of the nails) Usually affects toenails. Gnarled, thick and often long, curly nails.	Seek help from a chiropodist.
White flecks on nails Small white flecks on the nail that move up with the growing nail. 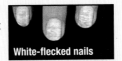 White-flecked nails	No treatment needed. It does not signify calcium deficiency (a common myth); there is no known cause.

Swollen ankles and lower legs

Swollen ankles and lower legs often feel heavy and look puffy. The causes listed here relate to the swelling of the two ankles and lower legs. When just one ankle and lower leg is affected, this is likely to be due to arthritis, varicose veins or injury; very rarely, it results from a tumour in the pelvis pressing on the veins of the leg.

OCCASIONAL CAUSES: severe obesity; pregnancy; abnormal swelling or growth within the pelvis, especially in the ovaries (a pelvic mass); cirrhosis; premenstrual syndrome; anaemia; drug reaction.
RARE CAUSES: angioneurotic oedema (fluid accumulation).

COMMON CAUSES	ACTION
Congestive heart failure Swelling worsens as the day goes by, often reduced in morning. Associated with shortness of breath on exertion; possible wheezy cough and phlegm.	See GP as soon as possible for assessment and treatment.
Osteoarthritis Morning stiffness, night pain common. Swelling worse when joint pain worse. Increasingly likely from age 50.	Take OTC anti-inflammatories or painkillers. See GP non-urgently.
Kidney disease (nephritis or nephritic syndrome) The hands may also be swollen. Urine may be unusually frothy, bloodstained. You feel generally unwell.	See GP urgently.
Venous insufficiency Common in immobile and elderly people. Swelling often reduced in the morning after lying down at night.	See GP non-urgently for confirmation.
Underactive thyroid (hypothyroidism) Gradual onset, associated with coldness, tiredness and feeling slowed down. Skin may feel dry, hair brittle.	See GP as soon as possible for assessment and possible blood test.

Deafness

Deafness is the complete or partial inability to hear. Before it is diagnosed, deafness in children may cause difficulties at home – parents may think the child is ignoring them – and at school, with poor school performance sometimes being the first sign. More than 8 million adults in the UK have some degree of deafness.

OCCASIONAL CAUSES: fluid in inner ear (Ménière's disease); burst eardrum (barotrauma); nerve disease (viral acoustic neuritis); large nasal polyps or tumour in the nasopharynx (airway behind the nose); drugs (eg streptomycin, gentamycin, or aspirin overdose).
RARE CAUSES: benign tumour (acoustic neuroma); vitamin B_{12} deficiency; multiple sclerosis.

COMMON CAUSES	ACTION
Ear wax Sense of blockage in the ear, usually painless; possible yellow discharge of liquefied wax. Deafness may be sudden.	Try warm olive oil drops twice daily for a week. If not improving, see your GP or practice nurse.
Middle ear infection (otitis media) Severe, throbbing earache. Sudden relief of pain followed by pus discharge indicates the eardrum has perforated. Deafness sudden.	If not improving within three days, see GP as soon as possible.
Ear canal infection (otitis externa) Severe earache, made worse on pulling outer ear. Common after seaside holidays and in swimmers. Deafness sudden.	See GP as soon as possible for antibiotic/antifungal eardrops. Reduce risk after swimming by washing ears out with boiled, cooled tap water.
Glue ear (secretory otitis media) A common painless childhood problem. Deafness is gradual.	See GP for examination and possible further investigation.
Noise damage to cochlea Onset of deafness very gradual and starts with loss of high-frequency tones. Most common in adults aged over 45.	See GP for examination and possible specialist referral.

Earache

Earache can affect just the inner ear canal or the outer ear (pinna) or both. It can start suddenly or gradually, can be mild or severe, hot, burning, throbbing, stabbing or dull. Referred pain from the throat or upper jaw may be felt in the ear, which shares the same nerve supply.

OCCASIONAL CAUSES: upper jaw joint dysfunction; dental abscess; impacted molar tooth; cranial nerve pain (trigeminal neuralgia); ear canal eczema or seborrhoeic dermatitis.
RARE CAUSES: inflammation behind ear (mastoiditis); arthritis of the neck (cervical spondylosis); benign wax-producing growth (cholesteatoma); cancer; burst eardrum.

COMMON CAUSES	ACTION
Middle ear infection (infective otitis media) Pain does not worsen on pulling external ear; possible ear discharge and fever. Deafness in affected ear.	Take paracetamol, but see GP if not improving after two days, or sooner if discharge appears.
Ear canal infection (infective otitis externa) Pain made worse on pulling external ear; discharge usually present. Possibly some deafness.	See GP as soon as possible for examination and treatment.
Boils of the ear canal and external ear Very painful and made worse by pulling external ear; possible discharge. Boils or acne elsewhere likely.	See GP as soon as possible for examination and antibiotic treatment.
Injury and foreign body (including wax) Deafness, pain on pulling outer ear and possible discharge. Common in toddlers and cotton-bud users.	Do not attempt removal. See GP for removal or referral to specialist.
Throat problems Pain made worse by swallowing. Swelling of glands in neck below jaw. Fever. The cause may be tonsillitis, pharyngitis or an abscess next to a tonsil (quinsy).	See GP for examination and treatment or referral (quinsy requires urgent surgery).

Eyes, red and painful

Eye pain can start suddenly or gradually, can be mild or severe, hot, burning, stabbing or dull and throbbing. All eye pain is serious and needs urgent treatment. By far the most common cause is infection, as in conjunctivitis; but if only one eye is affected other causes are more likely.

OCCASIONAL CAUSES: other inflammations (eg keratoconjunctivitis, affecting the cornea; episcleritis, soreness of the eyeball wall); collagen diseases (eg Reiter's syndrome, systemic lupus erythrematosus, ankylosing spondylitis, rheumatoid arthritis); injury such as a bruise or wound; chemical burns and arc eye, which affects welders; infection of the eyeball capsule (orbital cellulitis). **RARE CAUSES:** gout; granulomas – disorders associated with chronic inflammation (eg tuberculosis, sarcoidosis, toxoplasmosis); malignant tumour in the eye or invasion from tumour directly behind the nose.

COMMON CAUSES	ACTION
Acute conjunctivitis One or both eyes are red and sore, with sticky yellow or green discharge. Blurring of vision temporarily resolved when discharge is wiped away. 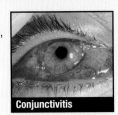 Conjunctivitis	If the eyelids are stuck together, bathe gently with clean, warm water; do not force lids apart. See GP urgently for treatment.
Acute iritis (inflammation of the iris) Vision is blurred. No discharge. Pupil in affected eye does not constrict in light, which hurts the eye.	See GP urgently: requires specialist referral.
Acute glaucoma (high pressure in eye) Blurred vision. The pupil is large and the cornea (the clear part of the front of the eye) may look hazy; eyeball feels hard and is very painful to touch. 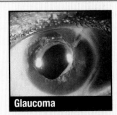 Glaucoma	See GP urgently: requires specialist referral.
Cornea inflammation (keratitis) or corneal ulcer A small grey patch may be seen on the clear part of the cornea (the front of the eye); possible discharge and blurred vision.	See GP urgently: requires specialist referral.
Corneal abrasion or superficial foreign body Impact from a blow or feeling of something getting into the eye is usually remembered. A bruise or foreign body may be visible.	Do not attempt removal. Cover eye and see GP urgently. If high-speed impact from a foreign body (eg a stone) may have occurred, go straight to casualty.

Gums, bleeding

Bleeding gums may be painful or not depending on the cause; the most common is gum infection as a result of poor dental hygiene. See a dentist first. If the cause is not dental, see a GP non-urgently for investigation.

OCCASIONAL CAUSES: aphthous mouth ulcers (the most common kind); herpes infection of mouth and gums (acute herpetic gingivostomatitis); autoimmune diseases; cancer in the mouth (oral neoplasia); blood abnormalities, especially acute myeloid leukaemia. **RARE CAUSES:** malabsorption; scurvy.

COMMON CAUSES	ACTION
Gingivitis (inflammation of the gums) or gum disease The gums are swollen and painful; the breath smells bad.	See dentist as soon as possible.
Pregnancy gingivitis During pregnancy the gums are swollen, but not painful; the breath does not smell bad.	See dentist as soon as possible.
Acute necrotizing ulcerative gingivitis Swollen, painful gums; foul breath; possible fever and feeling generally unwell.	See dentist as soon as possible, or urgently if feeling unwell.
Injury from poorly fitting dentures The cause is usually obvious from looking at the dentures and the sore part of the mouth.	See dentist to check fit of dentures.

Headache

A headache may be dull or sharp, constant or throbbing, aching or shooting, mild or severe. It is usually only a cause for concern if it lasts for several days or more, or is unusually severe. Many people fear it indicates a brain tumour, but this is extremely rare; tension and stress are easily the most common cause.

OCCASIONAL CAUSES: blood sugar deficiency; fatigue and/or sleep deprivation; nerve pain (eg trigeminal neuralgia); temporal arteritis (inflammation of the artery walls); post-concussional syndrome; drugs (eg nitrates). **RARE CAUSES:** cluster headache; brain tumour; meningitis (see page 28); intracerebral haemorrhage (bleeding into the brain); carbon monoxide poisoning (from a blocked boiler flue).

COMMON CAUSES	ACTION
Anxiety or depression The forehead or back of head may be sore to touch. Often described as feeling like a band around the head.	Take paracetamol for pain. Address causes of tension. If problematic, see GP non-urgently to discuss.
Sinus inflammation (frontal sinusitis) Throbbing pain over eyes made worse by stooping and coughing. Possible fever, green or yellow nasal catarrh.	Try steam inhalations, OTC painkillers, decongestants. If not improving within five days, see GP as soon as possible.
Migraine Severe throbbing headache, usually on one side of the head. Light hurts eyes; nausea, vomiting common. May be preceded by flashing lights or zigzag lines in vision.	Take OTC painkillers; rest in dark room (pain often disappears after a sleep). See GP non-urgently if recurrent; if attack very severe and lasting more than six hours, call for home visit.
Arthritis of the neck (cervical spondylosis) Pain is felt from the neck, up the back of the head, and to the top of the scalp; there is often a grating feeling in neck on turning. Common in people aged over 60.	Take OTC painkillers. If home treatment unsuccessful, see GP non-urgently.
Eyestrain Pain usually on one side, over or behind one eye. May happen after prolonged, concentrated reading.	See optician for eye test. Pace periods of reading with rest and looking at distant objects to relax eyes.

Hoarseness

With hoarseness the voice becomes quieter and huskier. It may occur with a sore throat or pain in the windpipe, depending on the cause. In general, if it slowly increases and persists it is of more concern than sudden hoarseness. See a GP if it lasts two weeks or more. Hoarseness with fever and unusual difficulty in breathing or sensation of swelling in the throat merits an urgent GP appointment.

OCCASIONAL CAUSES: inflammation of the gullet; benign tumours; rheumatoid arthritis of the voicebox; acute epiglottitis (throat inflammation); functional aphonia (loss of voice). **RARE CAUSES:** cancer of the larynx; chemical or physical damage.

COMMON CAUSES	ACTION
Inflammation of the air passage (acute viral laryngitis) Hoarseness starts suddenly after a sore throat or cold; it is usually painless by then.	Rest voice; it should return within a week. Steam inhalations and soothing drinks may help.
Voice overuse (shouting, screaming) The cause is obvious in an otherwise well person.	As for Inflammation of the air passage, above.
Underactive thyroid (hypothyroidism) Occurs gradually, and is associated with feeling cold, tired and slowed down. Skin may feel dry, hair brittle.	See GP as soon as possible for assessment and possible blood test.
Smoking May follow a sudden excess, for instance, after a party.	As for Inflammation of the air passage, above. Also, stop smoking.
Sinusitis (sinus inflammation) Fever and green or yellow nasal catarrh. Severe, dull pain above and/or below eyes on one or both sides, made worse on stooping.	As for Inflammation of the air passage, above, and use OTC decongestants. If pain not settling within five days, see GP for possible antibiotic treatment.

Mouth ulcers

An ulcer is a non-healing break in a body surface tissue. Mouth ulcers rarely need medical advice, but recurrent ulcers may signify an underlying problem; dentists are often best placed to investigate causes and treatments.

OCCASIONAL CAUSES: infection with coxsackie virus (eg herpangina – a throat infection, and hand-foot-and-mouth disease, which causes blisters; both affect young children); inflammatory bowel disease (eg ulcerative colitis, Crohn's disease); herpes simplex and herpes zoster; glandular fever; erosive lichen planus (an itchy skin disease).
RARE CAUSES: cancer; leukaemia; tuberculosis; Behçet's syndrome.

COMMON CAUSES	ACTION
Injury Often associated with a jagged tooth edge, an area inside the cheek getting bitten, or badly fitting dentures.	See dentist as soon as possible for assessment.
Recurrent aphthous ulceration The ulcers usually appear in crops, and recur. 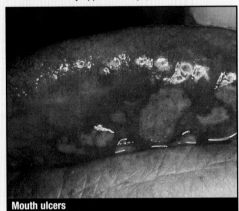 Mouth ulcers	See dentist as soon as possible for assessment.
Severe inflammation of the gums Medically known as acute necrotizing ulcerative gingivitis, this produces sore, bleeding gums with ulcers. The breath is foul.	See dentist urgently.
Thrush The inside of the mouth shows white patches that scrape off easily. In adults thrush may be associated with an underlying problem, such as diabetes. 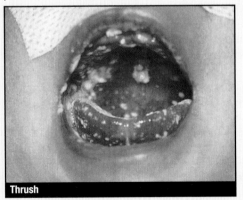 Thrush	See GP as soon as possible for assessment.
Anaemia (deficiency of iron, B_{12} or folic acid) The lips, tongue and inside of eyelids may look pale. The tongue may be sore, and there may be sores on the corners of the mouth.	See GP as soon as possible for assessment.

Neck stiffness, sudden

Neck stiffness is the sensation of tightness and pain in the neck on trying to move the head. Meningitis is a feared cause of neck stiffness but is extremely rare (see page 28). Its symptoms (headache, neck stiffness, dislike of bright light and meningism, see right) occur in any severe general bacterial infection. If in doubt, phone your GP.

OCCASIONAL CAUSES: exacerbation of rheumatoid arthritis; abscess in neck; psychological causes; intracerebral haemorrhage (bleeding into the brain); brain tumour.
RARE CAUSES: inflammation of the brain (meningitis); fracture of a vertebra; bone tumour; uncommon infections (eg tetanus, leptospirosis, psittacosis); brain abscess.

COMMON CAUSES	ACTION
Wry neck (acute torticollis) Often present from waking, or develops after a trivial twisting movement of neck. Turning head to one side is very painful; head often held twisted and to one side.	Take OTC painkillers, gently massage painful muscle. See GP urgently if pain relief is inadequate.
Exacerbation of pre-existing osteoarthritis All neck movements are painful. When the neck is moved a creaking or grating feeling and sound is common.	Take OTC anti-inflammatories or painkillers. See GP as soon as possible if these fail to work.
Viral nose or throat infection Glands in neck enlarged. Feeling unwell with mild fever. General aches and pains common.	Take paracetamol and cool drinks; rest. See GP if not settling within five days.
Whiplash injury Often happens after a road traffic accident. Increasing stiffness and pain over several days following an accident. May be troublesome for months afterwards.	Take OTC anti-inflammatories or painkillers. See GP if not helping. Physiotherapy may be useful.
Meningism Headache, neck stiffness, dislike of bright light. May be caused by infection, eg pneumonia. Severely ill with high fever. Many of the symptoms are the same as for meningitis (see page 28).	See GP urgently; if travel is impossible, ask for a home visit.

Nosebleed

Bleeding from the nose usually settles with simple first aid: sit in a chair with the head slightly forward; firmly pinch the nose between the bony part and the nostrils for ten minutes; do not blow the nose for at least three hours. If bleeding does not stop after an hour, go to casualty for treatment to stop the bleeding.

OCCASIONAL CAUSES: nasal septal granulomas (inflammatory lumps) and perforations of the septum; severe liver disease; cancers of nose, sinuses; abnormal anatomy (crooked nasal septum); injury.
RARE CAUSES: thrombocytopaenia (lack of blood-clotting cells); leukaemia; coagulation problems (eg haemophilia); deficiency of vitamin C or K.

COMMON CAUSES	ACTION
Spontaneous Sudden bleeding with no apparent cause. May be aggravated by nose-picking and sneezing. May recur.	Follow advice in introduction, left. See GP non-urgently if recurrent.
High blood pressure (hypertension); often with artery blockage (atherosclerosis) Nosebleeds come suddenly, with no apparent cause, and tend to be recurrent. Often associated with blockage of the arteries (atherosclerosis).	Follow advice in introduction, left. If you have hypertension, see GP as soon as possible for blood pressure check.
Nasal infection and ulceration Green nasal discharge and crusting usually already present; nose is painful inside.	Follow advice in introduction, left. See GP urgently for assessment.
Drug reactions Sudden bleeding with no apparent cause, and tends to be recurrent. Often associated with unexplained bruising on the body. May be a reaction to warfarin, aspirin or cytotoxic drugs.	Follow advice in introduction, left. See GP urgently for blood test to check blood clotting.
Inflammations of the nose (allergic or atrophic rhinitis) Nosebleeds recurrent, and associated with blocked nose.	Follow advice in introduction, left. See GP non-urgently for assessment.

Swallowing, difficulty in

This could be pain on starting to swallow, pain on swallowing, or the sensation of something in the throat when not swallowing. Anyone over the age of 60 complaining of difficulty in swallowing ought to be seen by a GP, especially if the person is unexpectedly losing weight.

OCCASIONAL CAUSES:
cancers (eg pharyngeal, bronchial and gastric carcinoma, lymphoma); oesophageal achalasia (muscle abnormality); abnormal dryness of the mouth (xerostomia).
RARE CAUSES: neurological problems (eg myasthenia gravis).

COMMON CAUSES	ACTION
Anxiety (globus hystericus) No difficulty in swallowing solids or liquids, but frequent sensation of something in the throat.	Try to deal with cause of stress. See GP non-urgently for examination and help with anxiety.
Inflammation of the gullet (reflux oesophagitis) Acid regurgitation on stooping and lying down. Heartburn after meals and with hot drinks. Nocturnal cough and foul taste in mouth are common.	Try OTC antacids. If needed, lose weight; wear loose clothing. Stop smoking. See GP non-urgently if this fails.
Narrowing of the oesophagus (benign peptic stricture) Difficulty in swallowing gradually gets worse. Heartburn and regurgitation of undigested food are possible.	See GP as soon as possible for investigation.
Cancer of the oesophagus, or gullet As for narrowing of the bowel above, but also with weight loss.	See GP as soon as possible for investigation.
Pharyngeal pouch Intermittent regurgitation of undigested food, hours after a meal. Swelling in neck possible.	See GP non-urgently for specialist referral.

Throat, sore

The pain of a sore throat may be dull or sharp, constant or throbbing, aching or shooting, mild or severe, depending on the cause. Viral infection is the cause in most cases; these will settle with simple home care, eg paracetamol, lozenges and cool drinks or ice cream. In general, if a sore throat is not showing signs of settling within five days, see a GP as soon as possible.

OCCASIONAL CAUSES:
thrush (oropharyngeal candidiasis); some forms of nerve pain (eg neuralgia); injury (foreign body or scratch from crispy food); acute ulcerative gingivitis; ulceration.
RARE CAUSES:
angina pectoris (cramping cardiac pain); oropharyngeal cancer (throat cancer at mouth level); retropharyngeal abscess (abscess in the tissues behind the throat).

COMMON CAUSES	ACTION
Viral pharyngitis (throat inflammation) Often follows a cold. Glands in neck may be enlarged. Feeling unwell with mild fever. General aches and pains common. Throat looks uniformly red but not swollen.	Take paracetamol, anaesthetic lozenges, cool drinks. If not settling in five days, see GP as soon as possible.
Tonsillitis streptococcal pharyngitis ('strep throat') Neck glands enlarged, painful. High fever; red spotty rash on body possible. Pus visible on red, swollen throat. Feeling very ill. Joints may be stiff and sore.	If pus clearly visible, and you are very unwell, see GP urgently.
Glandular fever (Epstein-Barr viral infection) Glands in neck and elsewhere (groins, armpits) swollen; tonsils show white patches. Rash may occur. Extreme tiredness possible for weeks after throat has improved.	See GP as soon as possible to confirm diagnosis (possible blood test) and plan recovery.
Quinsy (peritonsillar abscess) Extreme pain and visible swelling on one side of throat. The uvula, which hangs down at the back of the mouth, is pushed over to one side.	See GP urgently: this requires urgent surgery. If any difficulty in breathing, dial 999 or go straight to casualty.
Gullet inflammation (reflux oesophagitis) Often worse at night; a foul taste is often noted in the morning. Acid heartburn brought on by hot drinks and stooping. Acid may be tasted in the mouth on stooping.	Take OTC antacids. If overweight, lose weight; loosen clothing round waist. If a smoker, stop. See GP non-urgently if problem continues.

Tinnitus

Tinnitus sufferers perceive sounds that are not created outside the body; these may be low- or high-pitched, resembling many different noises.

OCCASIONAL CAUSES: chronic ear infection and glue ear (serous otitis media); a sudden loud noise; head injury; impacted wisdom teeth; drugs (eg aspirin overdose, loop diuretics, quinine); high blood pressure (hypertension), blocked arteries (atherosclerosis). RARE CAUSES: benign tumour (acoustic neuroma); severe anaemia and renal failure; spasm of the soft palate muscles (palatal myoclonus); anxiety.

COMMON CAUSES	ACTION
Ear wax Sudden onset of low-pitched noise; may be associated with dizziness and pain in the ear. Otherwise you feel well.	If no pain or previous perforation of eardrum, use OTC wax-removing drops to loosen wax. If this fails, see practice nurse for ear wash-out.
Hearing loss Gradual onset, may be low- or high-pitched noise. Associated with deafness on affected side. There is no dizziness.	See GP non-urgently.
Middle ear inflammation (suppurative otitis media) Sudden onset with severe pain, discharge and deafness on the same side. Fever may be present.	See GP urgently.
Middle ear bone overgrowth (otosclerosis) Very gradual onset with hearing loss in younger people. May be family history of otosclerosis.	See GP non-urgently.
Ménière's disease (inner ear disease) May be present all the time, but is worse at times of flare-ups, when sudden and disabling vertigo and nausea develop. Gradual hearing loss occurs.	See GP non-urgently, or urgently if vertigo is present.

Tongue, painful

Soreness often results when the tongue is accidentally bitten. This is a short-lived problem. For a serious injury to the tongue (which will bleed copiously), go straight to casualty. Longer-term cases should be looked at by a GP or dentist.

OCCASIONAL CAUSES: inflammation of the tongue (glossitis); burning mouth syndrome (psychological cause); fissured tongue (a tongue with cracks on the surface, usually painless); nerve pain (glossopharyngeal neuralgia); lichen planus (an itchy skin disease). RARE CAUSES: cancer of the tongue; drugs (eg mouthwashes, aspirin burns).

COMMON CAUSES	ACTION
Geographic tongue (erythema migrans) Red area with map-like border, slowly changing shape over weeks. It is long-term and gets worse with spicy/bitter foods.	See dentist as soon as possible for assessment.
Thrush (candida infection) Inside of mouth has white patches that scrape off easily. In adults, may be associated with underlying problem, such as diabetes, steroid treatment or taking antibiotics. 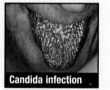 **Candida infection**	See GP as soon as possible for assessment.
Injury May be associated with a jagged tooth edge, the area inside the cheek getting bitten or burnt, or badly fitting dentures.	See dentist as soon as possible for assessment.
Anaemia (deficiency of iron, vitamin B_6 or B_{12}) The lips, tongue and inside of the eyelids may look pale and there may be sores on the corners of the mouth.	See GP as soon as possible for assessment.
Aphthous ulceration The ulcers usually appear in crops, and often recur. 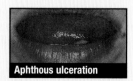 **Aphthous ulceration**	See dentist as soon as possible for assessment.

Abdominal pain: pregnancy

In the later stages of pregnancy, this could be labour. When a period has been missed, severe pain low in one side of the pelvis may represent an ectopic pregnancy (in which the fetus develops outside the uterus). In general, seek medical advice for abdominal pain in pregnancy, or vaginal bleeding with no pain.

OCCASIONAL CAUSES: constipation/irritable bowel syndrome; ectopic pregnancy; appendicitis; red degeneration of fibroid (a fibroid dies and fills with blood); twisting (torsion) and/or rupture of ovarian cyst or tumour. **RARE CAUSES:** twisting (torsion) and/or rupture of the uterus; inflammation of the gall bladder (cholecystitis); liver congestion caused by pre-eclampsia; blood within sheath of rectus muscle.

COMMON CAUSES	ACTION
Strain in symphysis pubis (joint within pubic bone) Severe pain around pubic bone, which is painful to the touch. Worse on standing and walking, relieved by rest.	Rest. Paracetamol is safe to use after the first three months.
Possible miscarriage Brisk vaginal bleeding with crampy, period-like pains. Affects 20–40 per cent of pregnancies in the first three months.	Take urgent GP advice or go straight to casualty.
Labour Very strong cramping pains, becoming longer and more frequent. Some 6 per cent of labours are premature.	Contact midwife, GP or labour ward for confirmation.
Placental abruption Torrential vaginal bleeding in late pregnancy, with severe lower abdominal pain, may indicate that the placenta has become detached from the wall of the uterus.	This is an emergency. Dial 999 and lie down until help arrives.
Kidney infection (pyelonephritis) Fever, frequent passing of small amounts of urine that may be foul and/or bloodstained. Severe, dull pain on one side of the back. More likely after 20 weeks and soon after delivery.	Urgent antibiotic treatment is needed. Contact GP urgently.

Abdominal pain: recurrent, adults

Recurrent pain along with weight loss or red blood in the faeces should prompt making a GP appointment. Jet-black faeces result from bleeding into the stomach; this emergency needs urgent hospital treatment.

OCCASIONAL CAUSES: gallstones; kidney obstruction (hydronephrosis); inflammatory bowel disease; inflammation of the gut (coeliac disease); nerve pain after herpes (post-herpetic neuralgia); spasms in the tubes draining the kidney (ureteric colic). **RARE CAUSES:** chronic pancreatitis (inflammation of the pancreas); subacute (intermittent) obstruction of the bowel (eg adhesions, cancer and diverticulitis); psychological abdominal pain.

COMMON CAUSES	ACTION
Irritable bowel syndrome (IBS) Bloating, crampy, colicky pains, relieved by passing wind or opening the bowels. There is often diarrhoea mixed with pellety faeces and mucus.	Often triggered by stress, so look for and address the cause. Symptoms can be helped by antispasmodics.
Recurrent urinary tract infection Frequent passing of small amounts of urine, often with stinging. Pain is felt low in the pelvis and back, or in one loin if a kidney is affected. Fever may be present.	See GP urgently: swift antibiotic treatment essential. May need later investigation.
Chronic peptic ulcer Continuous gnawing pain felt just under the breastbone. May be relieved by some foods, worsened by others.	Non-urgent GP appointment for investigation and treatment.
Constipation Hard faeces that are difficult to pass. Griping, colicky pain often felt on the left of the abdomen.	Increase fibre and fluid in diet, and level of activity, especially if elderly.
Infection of the alimentary tract (diverticulitis) Severe griping pains all over the abdomen; blood and mucus passed with diarrhoea. Fever.	See GP urgently for antibiotic treatment.

Abdominal pain: recurrent, children

Children may complain frequently of tummy aches, usually a vague and mild pain, felt in varying places in the abdomen. If this recurs over several months, parents should consult a GP. It is very rarely serious (unless it is caused by a urinary infection, which needs vigorous treatment to avoid kidney infection and scarring).

OCCASIONAL CAUSES: protein sensitivity (coeliac disease); parasites in gut; diabetes mellitus; obstruction in the kidney .
RARE CAUSES: sickle-cell disease; tuberculosis; temporal lobe epilepsy.

COMMON CAUSES	ACTION
Recurrent viral illnesses Coincides with a mild, feverish general illness.	Take paracetamol and fluids; rest during illness. Contact GP if significant interference with everyday life.
Abdominal migraine Caused by anxiety, depression or general unhappiness, there is rarely any noticeable illness. Poor school performance is common.	Arrange a non-urgent GP appointment.
Recurrent urinary infections Fever and painful, frequent urination.	Seek urgent GP advice. Needs antibiotics and usually further investigation.
Constipation Colicky or griping pain. May have overflow diarrhoea, when liquid contents of higher bowel bypass hard faeces.	Take plenty of fluids, eat a high-fibre diet, and exercise.
Food allergy Diarrhoea in an otherwise happy, healthy child.	No treatment. Identify and avoid the trigger food.

Abdominal pain: sudden, adults

Sudden, severe and unremitting abdominal pain in adults nearly always warrants an urgent GP examination. It can be felt in any part of the abdomen, or all over, and can have any character. Visit the surgery if possible, or ask for an urgent home visit.

OCCASIONAL CAUSES: gall bladder inflammation (cholecystitis); renal pain or ureteric colic from urinary stone; inflammation of the large intestine (diverticulitis); bowel obstruction (eg adhesions, carcinoma, strangulated hernia, volvulus); kidney infection (pyelonephritis).
RARE CAUSES: Crohn's disease and ulcerative colitis; pancreatitis; hepatitis; ischaemic bowel disease; dissecting or leaking aortic aneurysm; ketoacidosis in diabetics.

COMMON CAUSES	ACTION
Peptic ulcer Severe pain just below the solar plexus (breastbone). May be relieved by milky drinks or antacids.	See GP urgently, or ask for home visit.
Acute gastritis (inflammation of the stomach lining) Severe pain just below the solar plexus (breastbone). Vomiting usual.	See GP urgently, or ask for home visit.
Gallbladder or bile duct obstruction (biliary colic) Severe, griping pain just beneath bottom-right ribs. Bowel motions may be pale and urine dark.	See GP urgently, or ask for home visit.
Appendicitis Severe, constant pain in lower-right abdomen, often starting around the navel. Fever usually present. You may feel very ill, and may have vomiting and/or diarrhoea. Symptoms are similar in children.	See GP urgently. Do not eat or drink.
Gastroenteritis (stomach and intestine inflammation) Colicky pain anywhere in abdomen. Watery diarrhoea and vomiting.	Urgent GP telephone advice needed. Sip clear fluids (water, flat lemonade, diluted squash) even if vomiting.

Abdominal swellings

Most people experience abdominal swelling after certain foods, or too much food; the abdomen returns to normal within a day or two. Progressive swelling needs medical attention, especially if it is associated with weight loss.

OCCASIONAL CAUSES: build-up of fluid in the abdominal cavity (ascites); cancer of the colon (causing partial bowel blockage); ovarian mass (benign cyst or malignant tumours); cancer of the stomach; enlarged liver.
RARE CAUSES: cancer of the pancreas; enlarged spleen (splenomegaly); lymph node swelling around the aorta (para-aortic lymphadnopathy; kidney cysts and cancers.

COMMON CAUSES	ACTION
Pregnancy No periods for three months or more. Nausea and sore breasts may occur several weeks before abdominal swelling is noticed.	Use a home pregnancy test (now as reliable as hospital tests).
Irritable bowel syndrome (IBS) Diarrhoea, slimy or pelletty bowel motions, and wind. Frequent changes in size of abdomen. Colicky, griping abdominal pain.	Try a high-fibre diet. Deal with psychological stress (a common cause).
Constipation and wind Overflow diarrhoea, in which liquid contents of the higher bowel bypass hard faeces, may follow a period of constipation.	Try a high-fibre diet and exercise; laxatives may be useful in the short term. In elderly people, see GP if constipation is a new symptom, and laxative treatment fails.
Enlarged bladder (outflow obstruction) Thin, slow stream of urine; dribbling at end of stream.	Seek urgent GP advice. Bladder blockage must be relieved.

Anal pain

With pain, the anal ring of muscle (sphincter) goes into spasm; this can cause constipation, which in turn increases the pain. In general, this symptom needs to be seen by a GP, and promptly if accompanied by weight loss and/or change in frequency and consistency of bowel motions.

OCCASIONAL CAUSES: inflammation of alimentary tract (Crohn's disease); coccydynia (pain at end of spine); inflammation of the prostate gland (prostatitis); ovarian cyst or tumour.
RARE CAUSES: inflammation of the uterus lining (endometriosis); injury.

COMMON CAUSES	ACTION
Anal fissure Pain often starts during a bout of constipation; passing faeces is excruciatingly painful and there is often bleeding.	Use OTC anorectal anaesthetic creams liberally. Try a high-fibre diet to keep faeces soft. If not settling within a few days, see GP.
Thrombosed haemorrhoids and anal haematoma Both thrombosed haemorrhoids and anal haematoma result in a painful, hard lump or lumps on the anus.	As for Anal fissure, above; an ice pack and OTC oral painkillers may be helpful.
Abscess Swelling, bleeding and pus discharge all possible.	See GP urgently; may need surgery.
Muscle spasm (proctalgia fugax) Fleeting, intermittent, severe stabbing pain in rectum. May be associated with anxiety.	See GP non-urgently. Try OTC anorectal anaesthetics and prescribed antispasmodics.
Cancer of the anus and/or rectum Bleeding very likely; you may have a sense of rectal fullness even when no faeces are present.	See GP as soon as possible.

Constipation

Some people naturally open their bowels (defecate) several times a day, others only two or three times a week. Constipation is when defecation is less frequent, or if straining is ever needed. Weight loss and mucus or blood in the bowel motions occurring at the same time as constipation signifies the possibility of a serious problem.

OCCASIONAL CAUSES: chronic laxative use; underactive thyroid (hypothyroidism); cancer of the rectum or colon; dyschezia (long-term denial of the urge to open the bowels).
RARE CAUSES: tumours in the pelvis pressing on the colon; intestine inflammation (as in Crohn's disease) with stricture; in infants, Hirschprung's disease (a nerve disorder) and intestinal narrowing.

COMMON CAUSES	ACTION
Low-fibre diet and/or poor fluid intake More likely in people aged over 60, and children who are fussy eaters. Low fruit and vegetable content in diet.	Remedy dietary imbalance and increase daily fluid intake.
Inactivity Very likely in elderly people. Overflow diarrhoea often present: liquid contents of higher bowel bypass hard faeces.	Increase activity. If bedridden, abdominal massage can help.
Irritable bowel syndrome (IBS) Hard, pellety faeces interspersed with diarrhoea; often with mucus and painful colicky abdominal cramps. Bleeding is never present in IBS alone.	Increase dietary fibre. See GP non-urgently for antispasmodic treatment. Often triggered by stress: identify and remedy cause.
Painful anal conditions Often sudden onset and caused by, for example, anal fissure, haemorrhoids, abscess, florid warts. Attempts to defecate are excruciatingly painful. Blood may be present on paper or in the toilet pan, but not in the faeces.	Use OTC anal anaesthetic ointment and see GP as soon as possible, urgently if fever present (may be an abscess).
Drug treatments More likely in elderly people, and begins soon after starting drug treatment, such as opiates, iron, aluminium hydroxide, trycyclic antidepressants.	See GP for advice on change of treatment if possible.

Diarrhoea

Passing abnormally liquid and frequent faeces is very common; travellers have an increased risk of diarrhoea caused by food poisoning or tropical infection. People who work with food should not return to work until the diarrhoea has cleared and faeces have been tested for disease-causing organisms.

OCCASIONAL CAUSES: lactose intolerance; parasitic diseases (eg amoebiasis, giardiasis, hookworm); bowel neoplasm; inflammatory bowel disease (eg ulcerative colitis, Crohn's disease); excess alcohol.
RARE CAUSES: laxative misuse; excessive thyroid hormone (thyrotoxicosis); malabsorption (eg coeliac disease); allergy.

COMMON CAUSES	ACTION
Acute gastroenteritis Feeling ill; abdominal cramps and vomiting. Blood in the faeces not uncommon. May be caused by, for example, food poisoning, or infection by rotavirus.	Try OTC antidiarrhoeals/salt-replacement solutions. If fever, continuous pain or vomiting of 24 hours+, see GP urgently or ask for home visit. See GP as soon as possible if diarrhoea lasts 7 days+.
Antibiotic side effect Vomiting may also occur; should settle within a week after antibiotic treatment.	Telephone advice needed from GP about continuing antibiotics. May need a faeces test if it lasts more than a week after end of antibiotics.
Irritable bowel syndrome (IBS) Abdominal cramps, bloating, wind, diarrhoea, pellety faeces. Blood never present in IBS unless anus is inflamed.	Often stress-related: identify triggering cause. See GP for treatment/advice.
Diverticulitis (infection of the large intestine) Abdominal cramps, bloodstained diarrhoea. Constant pain and fever are serious signs.	Urgent GP appointment needed; request home visit if bedridden.
Overflow in constipation Previous constipation leading up to diarrhoea; abdominal cramps. Especially common in elderly people. Blood never present unless anus is inflamed.	Try OTC laxatives. If unsuccessful or problem recurs, see GP as soon as possible for examination.

Groin swellings

A swelling in the groin is unlikely to need urgent treatment, unless there is severe pain or general unwellness. A lump in the groin of a male with no testicle in the scrotum on that side suggests an undescended testicle; this should be surgically corrected.

OCCASIONAL CAUSES: abscess; cancer that has spread from elsewhere; hydrocele (fluid accumulation) in spermatic cord; low appendix mass; lipoma (a benign fatty tumour). **RARE CAUSES:** hip disease; lymphoma (malignant tumour); aneurysm (swelling on the femoral artery); neurofibroma (a benign tumour); undescended testis (especially in infants).

COMMON CAUSES	ACTION
Sebaceous cyst (blocked grease gland in skin) Hard lump within the skin itself. Usually no bigger than 1cm (⅓in), with a central dimple (punctum).	No immediate treatment needed unless troublesome; infection eventually likely, removal then necessary. See GP non-urgently.
Reactive lymph nodes (reaction to infection) Many lumps, variable in size, can be felt under the skin on either side of groin; these tend to come and go over a few weeks.	No treatment needed. This is simply a sign of a normal immunity, indicating that the lymph nodes are active.
Inguinal groin hernia Soft lump in the groin, appearing or getting bigger on coughing or straining. More common in men. 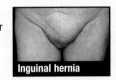 Inguinal hernia	See GP non-urgently, unless it becomes fixed, hard and painful: this may be a strangulated hernia, which is a surgical emergency.
Femoral hernia Similar to inguinal hernia but in the lower groin, and more common in women than men.	See Inguinal groin hernia, above.
Varicose vein in groin (saphena varix) Looks similar to a hernia but varicose veins are visible lower down the leg. Vibration felt on coughing and straining.	See GP non-urgently for surgical referral.

Rectal bleeding

Bleeding from the anus, on its own, or coating or mixed with bowel motions, is usually a result of constipation: this can cause haemorrhoids (which bleed), or tearing of the lining of the anal canal (anal fissure).

OCCASIONAL CAUSES: benign tumour (villous adenoma); injury; anticoagulant therapy; inflammatory bowel disease; cancer of the colon. **RARE CAUSES:** blood clotting disorders; blood vessel blockage in the bowel (ischaemic bowel disease); telescoping of bowel (intussusception); kidney failure (uraemia).

COMMON CAUSES	ACTION
Haemorrhoids (piles) Blood on paper and sometimes in toilet pan, as well as coating (but not mixed with) faeces. Possible soft and painless, or hard and painful, lumps on anus.	Take OTC haemorrhoidal ointments and laxatives. Have a high-fibre diet. See GP non-urgently for confirmation.
Anal fissure (tear of anal canal lining) Severe, tearing anal pain on passing hard faeces; then pain on passing normal faeces. Blood coating (not mixed with) faeces.	As for Haemorrhoids above, but see GP urgently if pain is severe.
Gastroenteritis (gut infection) Blood mixed with loose or liquid faeces. You may feel unwell; fever is likely if blood present. Colicky abdominal pain and sometimes vomiting.	Take OTC antidiarrhoeals and salt replacement solutions. If constant pain, fever or vomiting for 24 hours+, see GP urgently or ask for home visit.
Diverticulitis (infection of the large intestine) Abdominal cramps and bloodstained diarrhoea. Constant pain and fever are serious signs.	Urgent GP appointment needed; request home visit if bedbound.
Rectal cancer Bleeding, often painless and coating (but not mixed with) faeces. Possible constipation; sense of wanting to open bowels but no motions; mucus or discharge from the rectum.	See GP as soon as possible.

Rectal discharge

Rectal discharge may be identified by a mucus or pus discharge from the anus in the underwear. The main problem may be the resultant itchiness rather than the discharge itself or any dampness. The most common causes are benign, but it is a good idea to see a GP for this symptom to rule out the possibility of cancer.

OCCASIONAL CAUSES: rectal cancer; anal fistula (abnormal channel between rectum and anus allowing leakage); benign tumour (villous adenoma); inflammation of the alimentary tract (perianal Crohn's disease); ulcerative colitis is possible. **RARE CAUSES:** anal tuberculosis; anal cancer; syphilis; gonorrhoea; AIDS.

COMMON CAUSES	ACTION
Haemorrhoids (piles) Blood on toilet paper, sometimes in toilet pan, and coating (not mixed with) faeces. Soft painless or hard painful lumps may be felt on the anus, or emerge from it while passing faeces, which may be painful.	Take OTC haemorrhoidal ointments and laxatives; try a high-fibre diet. See GP non-urgently for confirmation.
Anal fissure (tear of anal canal lining) Severe tearing anal pain while passing hard faeces. Subsequent pain on passing faeces. Appearance of blood as for Haemorroids, above.	As for Haemorrhoids, above, but see GP urgently if pain severe.
Rectal prolapse Mucus discharge, possibly bloodstained. Rectum protrudes from anus while passing faeces.	See GP as soon as possible.
Rectal inflammation (proctitis) Intense pain in rectum, with mucus discharge, possibly mixed with pus and/or blood.	See GP urgently.
Perianal warts (condylomata acuminata) Cauliflower-like lumps around anus; pus discharge, possibly bloodstained. Passing faeces often painful, hygiene difficult.	Attend genito-urinary medicine clinic as soon as possible.

Vomiting, sudden

Vomiting is often preceded by a feeling of nausea. Blood in the vomit may have a serious cause, and require urgent medical advice. If vomiting is so severe that travel is impossible ask for a home visit. With a vomiting child, go to the surgery with a towel and a bowl or bucket: the wait is likely to be short.

OCCASIONAL CAUSES: low and high blood sugar (hypo- and hyperglycaemia); intestinal obstruction; kidney infection (pyelonephritis); calculus (stone in the ureter). **RARE:** peptic ulcer in adults, pyloric stenosis in infants (narrowing of lower outlet from stomach); meningitis (brain inflammation – see page 28); cerebral haemorrhage; bulimia nervosa; severe constipation.

COMMON CAUSES	ACTION
Gastroenteritis (gut infection) Also known as 'food poisoning': feeling ill; abdominal cramps and diarrhoea likely. Blood in the faeces not uncommon.	Take OTC antidiarrhoeals and salt-replacement solutions. If vomiting, fever or continuous pain continues for more than 24 hours, see GP urgently.
Inner ear inflammation (acute viral labyrinthitis) Sudden, severe vomiting and continuous vertigo; associated general viral illness, such as cold. Sensation of sounds in the ears or head (tinnitus) may be present.	See GP urgently; ask for home visit if travel is not possible.
Upper respiratory infection with marked coughing Most common in children, cough, cold or sore throat symptoms are usually present for a day or two before the vomiting, which occurs only with prolonged coughing bouts.	Try OTC decongestants and aromatic oils. Frequent sips of non-milky drinks. See GP urgently if not settled in a day.
Pregnancy Late, missed period. Nausea and sore breasts may occur several weeks before abdominal swelling is noticed.	Consult a home pregnancy test, now as reliable as hospital tests.
Appendicitis and other causes of acute pain Severe, continuous abdominal pain. Possible fever and diarrhoea; you may feel very ill. The abdomen may feel rigid, and movement may be very painful.	See GP urgently.

Breast lumps

A lump that changes in size over time is very unlikely to be cancer. But lumps appearing after the menopause and lumps causing skin dimpling or alterations in breast size or shape, or the direction of the nipple, should always be investigated for the possibility of cancer. Not all lumps require immediate specialist referral, but most GPs now have access to fast-track breast lump clinics.

OCCASIONAL CAUSES:
duct ectasia (dilation of the mammary ducts); lipoma (benign tumour); multiple cysts.
RARE CAUSES:
tuberculosis; sarcoma (malignant tumour); lymphoma; phylloides tumour (benign).

COMMON CAUSES	ACTION
Cyst The lump is smooth and firm, and may change with your menstrual cycle.	See GP as soon as possible.
Abscess Sudden onset of a hot, painful lump with fever and general feeling of illness.	See GP as soon as possible.
Fibroadenoma (benign lump) Smooth, round, very mobile lump.	See GP urgently. May need referral to hospital for incision under anaesthetic.
Breast tissue change (fibrous dysplasia) Affects both breasts: they feel generally lumpy rather than having individual lumps. May be painful and change with your periods.	See GP as soon as possible for confirmation. Referral may be worthwhile.
Cancer The lump is hard and irregular, and fixed to surrounding tissues. See introduction for suspicious features.	See GP routinely for confirmation and treatment.

Breast pain

Breast pain may be dull or sharp, constant or throbbing, aching or shooting, mild or severe, depending on the cause. Like breast lumps, breast pain often raises fear of the possibility of cancer. This is not a common cause, and it is unusual for pain to be the first sign of the disease: a lump would probably have been noticed already. Pain on one side, with a rash on the side of the chest or back (slightly higher than the breast) may be shingles (see page 27).

OCCASIONAL CAUSES:
cancer; onset of puberty; simple cyst; injury; lactation.
RARE CAUSES: tuberculosis; (angina); arthritis of the neck (cervical spondylosis); thrombophlebitis (inflammation of the vein); shingles.

COMMON CAUSES	ACTION
Pregnancy One of the earliest signs of pregnancy in a woman who has missed a period. Occurs on both sides. Morning sickness may be present.	If in doubt, get a home pregnancy test (now as accurate as hospital tests). If positive, see GP to discuss.
Menstrual breast pain (cyclical mastalgia) Both breasts become lumpy and tender as the menstrual period becomes due. Can be very sore.	See GP non-urgently to discuss treatment options.
Cracked or inflamed nipple Common in breastfeeding women. May affect one or both nipples or there may be reddening around the nipple on an otherwise normal breast.	Pharmacists and midwives can advise on OTC creams and ointments. Do not stop breastfeeding.
Mastitis (breast infection) One breast is excruciatingly painful and hot. There is reddening of a wedge-shaped area of skin, spreading out from the nipple. Fever is often present. Most common in pregnant or breastfeeding women.	Requires antibiotics. See GP urgently to reduce the risk of abscess formation. Do not stop breastfeeding.
Breast abscess Follows mastitis, sometimes even if treated with antibiotics. Signs as for mastitis, see above, with a hard and very painful lump under the inflamed area.	See GP urgently for hospital referral: requires incision under anaesthetic.

Intercourse, painful in women

Dryness and discharge are just two possible contributory factors to painful intercourse in women. It is a common problem and doctors have much experience in dealing with it; so do not hesitate to seek help.

OCCASIONAL CAUSES: repair of perineum following childbirth; fibroids in uterus; retroverted uterus; pelvic adhesions caused by previous surgery or infection; cystitis; urethritis.

RARE CAUSES: large ovarian cyst or tumour; urethral caruncle (fleshy protrusion); unruptured hymen; anal fissure (tear); thrombosed haemorrhoids (piles filled with clotted blood); perianal abscess.

COMMON CAUSES	ACTION
Vaginismus (spasm and dryness) The vagina is dry on attempting intercourse, and feels tight and too small inside. No pain otherwise; no discharge; normal periods. Psychological cause.	See GP non-urgently to rule out other causes and discuss best approach. Psychosexual therapy can be helpful.
Superficial infection Copious discoloured vaginal discharge that may smell unpleasant. Soreness and itching all the time. Pain from start of penetration. May be caused by bacterial or fungal vaginosis, ulceration or bartholinitis.	See GP urgently for assessment.
Menopausal vaginal dryness (atrophic vaginitis) Gradually increasing difficulty with intercourse. No vaginal discharge. Possible symptoms of menopause, unless already over. Pain from start of penetration.	See GP non-urgently for assessment. If bleeding has occurred, see GP as soon as possible.
Endometriosis (uterus lining tissue at other sites) Heavy, painful periods. Pain on deep intercourse.	See GP as soon as possible for assessment.
Pelvic inflammatory disease (PID) Pain on deep intercourse. Discharge and heavy and painful periods often present.	See GP as soon as possible for assessment.

Pelvic pain, chronic

Pelvic pain is said to be chronic if it has been present for three or more menstrual cycles, either around the time of the periods or throughout the menstrual cycle. The most frequent causes are gynaecological, and a GP might refer you to a gynaecologist.

OCCASIONAL CAUSES: recurrent urinary tract infection; mechanical low back pain (recurrent strain); uterovaginal prolapse; benign tumours (eg ovarian cyst, fibroids); chronic interstitial cystitis.

RARE CAUSES: cancers (eg of the ovary, cervix, bowel); inflammation of alimentary tract (diverticulitis); inflammatory bowel disease; subacute intermittent bowel obstruction; 'forgotten' intrauterine contraceptive device (coil).

COMMON CAUSES	ACTION
Endometriosis (uterus lining tissue at other sites) Often worse around periods, which are often heavy. Painful intercourse.	See GP non-urgently.
Chronic pelvic inflammatory disease (PID) Pain usually throughout the month; may be worse during periods, which are heavy. Difficulty conceiving.	See GP non-urgently.
Pelvic congestion Worse around periods, which are heavier than usual. Usually no problems during the rest of the month.	See GP non-urgently.
Irritable bowel syndrome (IBS) May be worse around periods, which are not heavier than usual. Abdominal bloating, colicky pain, diarrhoea, pelletly bowel motions and mucus. Urgent need to open bowels after eating, which often relieves pain.	See GP non-urgently.
Mid-cycle or ovulation pain, period pain Mid-cycle pain is short-lived and felt on one side, occurring 14 days after first day of last period. Period pain is usually just before and in first few days of period.	See GP non-urgently.

Pelvic pain, severe and sudden

Sudden, severe pain felt in the lower abdomen and in the pelvis is mostly felt by women. If the pain is so severe that travel is not possible, ask your GP for a home visit.

OCCASIONAL CAUSES: pelvic abscess; endometriosis (uterus lining tissue at other pelvic sites); prostatitis (in men); psychosexual factors.
RARE CAUSES: misplaced coil (intrauterine contraceptive device) leading to perforated uterus; referred pain (eg from spinal tumour, bowel spasm); rectal inflammation (proctitis); invasive cancer of ovaries or cervix; degeneration of fibroids.

COMMON CAUSES	ACTION
Acute pelvic inflammatory disease (PID) Pain is constant and severe; it may be felt in the back, and be worse on deep intercourse. Discoloured and/or bloodstained vaginal discharge. Fever; feeling unwell.	See GP urgently for assessment.
Urinary tract infection Low, deep, dull, constant pain, often in the back or higher on one side. Urgent desire to pass urine, but only small quantities passed (with burning pain). Urine may be smelly and/or bloodstained. Fever; feeling unwell.	See GP urgently for assessment.
Miscarriage After a missed period, crampy low pain like a bad period pain. Vaginal bleeding, ranging from a little brown discharge to copious red blood with clots.	Call GP for advice. Wear pad and save any solid material passed.
Ectopic pregnancy (development of fetus outside the uterus) Around two weeks after a missed period, severe crampy or constant pain on one side of the pelvis. Pain is followed by vaginal bleeding, possible serious haemorrhage.	See GP urgently for assessment. If vaginal bleeding has begun, dial 999.

Periods, absent

This refers to periods that have stopped in a previously menstruating woman; periods that never started are referred to as 'delayed puberty' (see page 63). Absent periods are not dangerous, but it is worth seeing a GP to treat the underlying causes.

OCCASIONAL CAUSES: under- or overactive thyroid (hypo- and hyperthyroidism); anorexia nervosa; severe general illness of any kind; excessive exercise or training; adrenal disorders (eg Addison's or Cushing's disease, congenital adrenal hyperplasia).
RARE CAUSES: prolactinoma (benign tumour causing over-production of the hormone prolactin); other pituitary tumours.

COMMON CAUSES	ACTION
Pregnancy Tender breasts, morning sickness; abdominal swelling after 10–12 weeks.	Try a home pregnancy test, as reliable as hospital tests. See GP if positive.
Physiological factors Causes might include breastfeeding, rapid weight loss or severe emotional stress. Absent periods may be associated with depression.	See GP non-urgently for investigation of weight loss or advice on stress.
Menopause (and premature ovarian failure) Hot flushes, night sweats, and sometimes unpredictable mood swings.	See GP non-urgently for investigation and to discuss available treatments.
Polycystic ovary syndrome (hormonal disorder) Often to some degree overweight, excess body hair and acne.	See GP non-urgently for investigation and possible specialist referral.
Drug treatment Possible milky breast discharge, for example, caused by: phenothiazines, metoclopramide, sodium-valproate, cytotoxics.	See GP non-urgently.

Periods, heavy

A period is heavy if bleeding is heavier or longer than the woman thinks it should be. A single heavy period can be caused by emotional upset or excessive exercise, so it is best to wait three cycles to establish a pattern before making a non-urgent GP appointment. (For causes of bleeding outside of periods, see page 63, Vaginal bleeding, irregular.)

OCCASIONAL CAUSES: puberty; menopause; intrauterine contraceptive device (coil); chronic pelvic inflammatory disease (PID); overactive thyroid (hyperthyroidism). **RARE CAUSES:** adrenal disorders and excess prolactin; liver disease; endometrial cancer.

COMMON CAUSES	ACTION
Dysfunctional uterine bleeding Periods are heavy but usually painless; the interval between them may be longer than usual. Otherwise you are well.	See GP urgently after three heavy periods.
Cervical or endometrial polyps (benign growths) Heavy periods may be painful; possible bleeding between periods and after intercourse.	See GP urgently after three heavy periods; or sooner if there is bleeding between periods or after intercourse.
Endometriosis (uterus lining tissue at other sites) Heavy periods are generally very painful. Intercourse may be painful; pain in pelvis may persist through the cycle.	See GP urgently after three heavy periods.
Fibroids (benign growths) Heavy periods may be painful. Possible pressure symptoms may be felt: discomfort during intercourse; need to empty bladder frequently and, very occasionally, leg swelling.	See GP urgently after three heavy periods.
Underactive thyroid (hypothyroidism) Heavy, sometimes irregular periods; associated with tiredness, feeling cold and slowed down. Weight gain, dry skin, brittle hair.	See GP urgently after three heavy periods, sooner if associated symptoms have already developed.

Periods, painful

Period pain (dysmenhorroea) is felt in the lower abdomen and back and is not always associated with heavy periods. Half of all the women in the UK have moderately painful periods; and more than ten per cent have severe pain. Painful periods developing later in life are usually treatable.

OCCASIONAL CAUSES: ovarian cysts (caused by endometriosis); abnormally positioned (retroverted) uterus; inflammation of the cervix (cervicitis); endometrial polyp (benign growth). **RARE CAUSES:** uterine malformation; unbroken hymen; defective development of uterus (hypoplasia); narrowing of the cervix (cervical stenosis); psychological factors.

COMMON CAUSES	ACTION
Primary dysmenorrhoea Pain starts with the first-ever period. Crampy pain is felt in the first few days of the period.	Take OTC painkillers or anti-inflammatories. See GP non-urgently if not settled after first six months, or if especially severe.
Endometriosis (uterus lining tissue at other sites) Pain often not crampy, and may be widespread through lower abdomen. Associated with deep pain on intercourse.	See GP non-urgently for examination and specialist referral for investigations.
Chronic pelvic inflammatory disease (PID) Deep pain felt on intercourse. Pain in pelvis may continue in rest of month. Follows an initial pelvic infection.	See GP non-urgently for examination and possible specialist referral.
Fibroids (benign growths) Progressively more painful periods, sometimes becoming increasingly heavy. Possible pressure symptoms including frequent passing of urine.	See GP non-urgently for examination and investigations.
Intrauterine contraceptive device (coil) Crampy pains felt during periods, which may be heavier than before coil is fitted.	See GP non-urgently to consider coil removal and alternative contraception.

Vaginal discharge

A certain amount of clear mucal discharge from the vagina is normal. Its thickness varies through the menstrual cycle. If it becomes coloured, offensive or excessive, it can be considered abnormal. In all cases, attend a genito-urinary medicine clinic if there is a possibility of a sexually transmitted disease.

OCCASIONAL CAUSES: cervical erosion (overgrowth of cells from the inner cervix); cervical polyp (benign growth); lost tampon, or other foreign body; intrauterine contraceptive device (coil); Bartholinitis (inflammation of glands at vaginal entrance). **RARE CAUSES:** cancer (eg vulval, vaginal, cervical, uterine); benign growth (fibroid).

COMMON CAUSES	ACTION
Excessive normal secretions Clear mucus discharge. May cause external discomfort through continuous dampness. You feel otherwise well.	See GP non-urgently.
Thrush (candida infection) Intense vaginal itching and soreness. There may be pain on passing urine. White, creamy, usually inoffensive discharge.	Take OTC thrush treatment. Your sexual partner, who may have no symptoms, should do the same. See GP if this fails.
Bacterial vaginosis Offensive yellow or greenish discharge. Vagina is usually not sore or itchy.	See GP as soon as possible.
Trichomonal vaginosis Offensive, often fishy-smelling, greyish, frothy discharge. The vagina is sore and itchy.	See GP as soon as possible.
Inflammation of the cervix (cervicitis) Caused by, for example, gonococcus, chlamydia or herpes. The discharge may be yellow or greenish, possibly offensive. Pain on deep intercourse. Vagina may be sore and/or itchy.	Attend genito-urinary medicine clinic as soon as possible. Refrain from sex until treatment is complete.

Vulval irritation

Irritation of the vulva results in itching and soreness. The vulva is made up of the inner and outer lips (labia) of the vagina and the space between them. The causes of vulval irritation may also affect the vagina.

OCCASIONAL CAUSES: inflammation from incontinence (ammoniacal vulvitis); psoriasis; lichen planus (an itchy skin disorder); infestations (eg, scabies, pubic lice); underlying psychosexual problem. **RARE CAUSES:** cancer; general disorders causing itching.

COMMON CAUSES	ACTION
Thrush (candida infection) Intense vaginal itching and soreness. Possible pain on passing urine. White, usually inoffensive, creamy discharge.	Take OTC thrush treatment. The same for your sexual partner, who may have no symptoms. See GP if this fails.
Bacterial or trichomonal vaginosis **Bacterial:** offensive yellow or greenish discharge; vagina usually not sore or itchy. **Trichonomal:** offensive, often fishy-smelling, greyish, frothy discharge; vagina is sore and itchy.	See GP as soon as possible or attend a genito-urinary medicine clinic.
Insufficient lubrication during intercourse Sore, possibly itchy vagina. Difficulties with intercourse are usually known already.	Ensure adequate foreplay; use a water-based lubricant gel. See GP non-urgently if problem persists.
Reactions to chemicals Sore, itchy vagina; usually no discharge. Otherwise you feel well. May be caused by bubble baths, feminine-hygiene douches or detergents.	Try OTC hydrocortisone cream; avoid offending product if identified. See GP as soon as possible if not better in five days.
Atrophic vaginitis Around or after the menopause, a sore (not itchy) vagina, with thin, dry and reddened lining of vulva and vagina. No discharge. Difficulties with intercourse.	As for Insufficient lubrication (see above). Discuss hormone replacement therapy (HRT) with GP.

Vulval swellings

A swelling or lump may develop in the vulva (the inner and outer lips of the vagina and the space between them), or originate elsewhere and become displaced into the vulva.

OCCASIONAL CAUSES:
varicose vein; dilated veins (varicocele); benign tumours (eg lipoma); prolapses of the uterus, bladder, rectum or bowel; urethral protuberance (caruncle); cervical polyp (benign growth). **RARE CAUSES:** cancer; traumatic haematoma (blood clot in tissue).

COMMON CAUSES	ACTION
Boil Solitary, painful, pus-filled spot which eventually bursts. It may not heal easily without treatment.	See GP urgently.
Sebaceous cyst (blocked grease gland in skin) Firm or hard lump fixed to the skin, and with a central hole or dimple (punctum).	Do not squeeze the cyst: this could cause painful inflammation. See GP non-urgently. No treatment is needed unless the cyst is causing problems.
Viral warts (condylomata acuminata) Crops of hard whitish or brown lumps appear anywhere on the surface skin of the vulva.	Attend a genito-urinary medicine clinic as soon as possible.
Bartholin's cyst (infected abscess) A painless, firm lump is felt in the lower vulva, under the skin on one side. There is no swelling in the surrounding area.	See GP non-urgently, or urgently if it becomes painful.
Inguinal groin hernia (protrusion) Swelling, usually in one groin, which may extend right into the outer lip (labium major). Increases in size on coughing. More common in smokers, women with chronic cough, and heavy manual workers.	See your GP non-urgently. If the lump cannot be pushed back into the abdomen and it becomes hard and painful, see GP urgently: it may result in possible strangulation of the hernia.

Vulval ulceration and sores

Ulcers and sores are non-healing breaks in a body surface tissue. Consult a doctor about any that appear on the vulva. If there is any possibility of a sexually transmitted disease, attend a genito-urinary medicine clinic and refrain from intercourse meanwhile.

OCCASIONAL CAUSES:
Bowen's and Paget's diseases; sexually transmitted diseases (eg lymphogranuloma venereum); diabetic and mycotic vulvitis (inflammation of the vulva); cancer. **RARE CAUSES:** syphilis; Behçet's syndrome; tuberculosis.

COMMON CAUSES	ACTION
Herpes simplex May cause fever and leave you feeling unwell. Crops of blister-like spots develop, becoming pus-filled then painful with scabs. Glands in groin are enlarged. Passing urine can be very painful; catheterization in hospital may be necessary.	Attend a genito-urinary medicine clinic urgently.
Excoriated (badly scratched) thrush (candida infection) Intense vaginal itching and soreness. There may be pain on passing urine. White, creamy discharge.	Take OTC thrush treatment. Your sexual partner should do the same, even if without symptoms. See a GP if this fails.
Abnormal tissue development (vulval dysplasia) Gradual onset of an itchy sore; no accompanying discharge; otherwise you feel well. Most common after the menopause.	See GP as soon as possible.
Squamous cell cancer An itchy, crusty lump gradually enlarges; no discharge.	See GP as soon as possible.
Excoriated (badly scratched) scabies A furiously itchy rash appears, often starting on the hands and spreading. It gets worse at night.	Try OTC antiscabies lotions; itch may last ten days after the treatment ends. It is contagious by direct contact only.

Breast swelling in men

In men, swelling of breast tissue can be felt behind the nipple area. For causes of lumps in women's breasts, see page 51. The causes are important, so a checkup is advisable.

OCCASIONAL CAUSES: hypothyroidism (underactive thyroid); chronic renal failure; testicular or adrenal cancer; cryptorchidism (undescended testicle), hypogonadism (underactivity of testes) and other causes of impaired testicular function.
RARE CAUSES: acromegaly (a growth hormone disorder); Klinefelter's syndrome (a genetic disorder in which male has one or more extra X chromosomes).

COMMON CAUSES	ACTION
Puberty Breast swelling often occurs on one side only during puberty. Other causes are very rare at this age.	If it has not settled on its own within three months, see GP non-urgently.
Drugs Both sides swollen; may be feeling generally unwell. Causes include use of spironolactone, cimetidine, digoxin, cyproterone, marijuana.	See GP as soon as possible.
Chronic liver disease Affects both sides. If the cause is alcohol-related, there may be other signs of alcohol excess, for example, red face and palms, weight loss, erratic behaviour and drunkenness.	See GP non-urgently for checkup and advice. Contact local drugs and alcohol agency for long-term help.
Lung cancer Affects both sides. Possible cough, shortness of breath, weight loss, coughing up blood. Rare in non-smokers.	See GP as soon as possible for assessment.
Hyperthyroidism (overactive thyroid) Affects both sides. Feeling unwell, anxious. Possible weight loss, fast pulse, sweaty skin, tremor of hands.	See GP as soon as possible for investigation and treatment.

Impotence

This is failure to achieve a normal erection; either a full erection dwindles before orgasm or it cannot be reached for any length of time. It may have a psychological cause, especially if a good morning erection is regularly achieved. Erections that dwindle after a set period are more likely to have a physical cause.

OCCASIONAL CAUSES: diabetic nerve damage; injury to the penis; post-prostate surgery; anatomical (eg phimosis – tightness of the foreskin); smoking; Peyronie's disease (causing the penis to bend during erection).
RARE CAUSES: impaired testicular function; blood clot (thrombosis); neurological disorders (eg multiple sclerosis); spinal cord compression (caused by tumour).

COMMON CAUSES	ACTION
Depression or anxiety Low mood, difficulty in sleeping, tearfulness, loss of confidence, all for two weeks or more.	See GP as soon as possible for assessment and treatment.
Excessive alcohol intake Red face and palms. Morning erections infrequent.	Seek help from a local drug and alcohol agency.
Relationship dysfunction Occasional failure to get an erection; good morning erections are usual.	Seek help from a specialist counselling service such as Relate.
Blood vessel problems Erection failure every time. Morning erections infrequent or absent. Cold legs or feet common. Possible causes are arterial insufficiency and excessive venous drainage.	See GP as soon as possible, especially if your legs or feet are cold.
Medication Erection failure every time. Morning erections infrequent or absent. May be caused by, for example, prostate cancer treatments, hypotensives, some antidepressants, spironolactone.	See GP as soon as possible for a review of your medication.

Penile pain

It is important to seek medical advice as soon as possible for penile pain, even if the pain is occasional, and especially if blood is passed painlessly in the urine. If there is no discharge, pain in the penis is unlikely to be caused by a sexually transmitted disease.

OCCASIONAL CAUSES:
herpes simplex; cancer (eg bladder, prostate); injury (eg zipper injury, urethral injury or foreign body); acute cystitis; anal fissure or inflamed haemorrhoid (pile).
RARE CAUSES: cancer of the penis, rectum and/or anus; Peyronie's disease (pain usually on erection); shingles (herpes zoster).

COMMON CAUSES	ACTION
Balanitis (fungal or bacterial infection of tip of penis) Usually a problem only in uncircumcised men; pus discharge from under the foreskin and painful tip of penis (glans penis). Passing urine may be painful.	See GP urgently.
Prostatic abscess, inflammation (prostatitis) Possible discharge from urethra (opening in end of penis), pain on passing urine. Severe, dull, rectal pain. Fever possible.	See GP urgently.
Urinary stone (calculus) Excruciating pain lasting minutes or hours; may begin on one side of abdomen or back. There may be blood in the urine.	See GP as soon as possible. Sieve urine through a tea strainer to catch stones; retain them to show to your GP.
Inflammation of the urethra (acute urethritis) Continual discharge from urethra with burning pain on passing urine. Fever and joint pains may also occur.	Consult a genito-urinary medicine clinic as soon as possible; until then abstain from all sexual intercourse.
Tight foreskin (phimosis) Difficulty and pain on passing urine through the tight opening in the foreskin, which may balloon during urination. Possible accompanying discharge from under the foreskin.	See GP as soon as possible.

Penile sores and ulceration

Sores and ulcers are non-healing breaks in a body surface tissue. Like penile pain, these symptoms often raise the fear of sexually transmitted disease or cancer. Cancer is a rare cause; sexually transmitted disease is much more likely. If this is a realistic possibility, refrain from all sexual intercourse until seen as soon as possible in a genito-urinary medicine clinic.

OCCASIONAL CAUSES:
shingles (herpes zoster); inflamed glans penis (balanitis circinata caused by Reiter's syndrome); sexually transmitted diseases (eg lymphogranuloma venereum).
RARE CAUSES: primary syphilis (chancre: painful sore); tertiary syphilis (gumma: painless soft tumour); penile cancer.

COMMON CAUSES	ACTION
Herpes simplex Crops of blister-like spots that become pus-filled and break down to a painful scab. Glands in groin enlarged. May have fever and be feeling unwell.	Attend a genito-urinary medicine clinic urgently; until then abstain from all sexual intercourse.
Boil/infected sebaceous cyst (blocked grease gland) Solitary, painful pus-filled spot that bursts and may not heal easily without treatment.	See GP urgently.
Warts, condylomata acuminata Crops of hard whitish or brown lumps appear on the surface of the skin, usually at the tip of the penis (glans penis).	Attend a genito-urinary medicine clinic as soon as possible; until then abstain from all sexual intercourse.
Balanitis (fungal or bacterial infection of tip of penis) Usually occurs in uncircumcised men only; pus discharge from under foreskin and painful tip of penis (glans penis). Passing urine may be painful.	See GP urgently.
Injury Injury (eg a zipper injury) is usually obvious. When torn, the frenulum (the bowstring-like thread joining the underside of the penis tip to the penis shaft) often bleeds dramatically.	See GP urgently or go to casualty. To stop any bleeding, apply firm pressure with a clean pad to the bleeding point.

Scrotal swellings

Swellings in the scrotum can affect males of all ages. Testicular cancer is rare, but is most common in the 20–40 age group. All men should practise self-examination of their scrotums at least once a month. See a GP as soon as possible if a lump is discovered.

OCCASIONAL CAUSES: torsion (twisting) of the testis; infection after surgery or catheterization; haematocele (blood-filled swelling); varicocele (dilated veins); congestive heart failure.
RARE CAUSES: testicular cancer (seminoma, teratoma).

COMMON CAUSES	ACTION
Inguinal (groin) hernia Swelling usually in one groin and descending towards scrotum; increases in size on coughing. Most common in smokers, men with chronic cough, and heavy manual workers.	See GP non-urgently, more quickly if lump cannot be pushed back into abdomen and is hard and painful.
Sebaceous cyst (blocked grease gland in skin) Firm or hard lump fixed to the skin, with a central hole or dimple (punctum).	Do not squeeze: may make it inflamed. No treatment needed unless causing problems. See GP non-urgently.
Hydrocele (fluid accumulation) Soft, painless swelling around one testicle.	See GP as soon as possible for confirmation.
Epididymal cyst Firm, round swelling at end of one testicle. Usually (but not always) painless.	See GP as soon as possible for confirmation.
Epididymo-orchitis (genito-urinary infection) One or both testicles are painful and swollen. You may feel generally unwell, with fever. The infection is sexually transmitted.	See GP urgently.

Testicular pain

When it occurs suddenly, testicular pain is usually excruciating and severe, and is likely to be caused by an urgent problem. A dull, dragging pain suggests a longer-term or less urgent problem. Testicular pain can occur in males of all ages.

OCCASIONAL CAUSES: varicocele (dilated veins); haematocele (blood-filled swelling); hydrocele (fluid-filled swelling); injury (fractured testis); undescended or misplaced testis.
RARE CAUSES: testicular cancer (seminoma, teratoma); syphilis; referred pain from spinal tumours.

COMMON CAUSES	ACTION
Acute orchitis (inflammation of the testes) Both sides affected; testicles painful to touch. Onset over a few hours. Generally feeling unwell, with fever. Glands in armpits, neck, groins may be enlarged and tender. Underlying cause may be mumps or, less commonly, flu or scarlet fever.	Take regular paracetamol. See GP urgently for diagnosis.
Acute epididymo-orchitis (genito-urinary infection) Onset over a few hours; usually both testicles painful. Supporting the testicles helps. Fever uncommon; possible discharge, frequent and painful passing of urine. Infection is sexually transmitted.	See GP urgently. Attend genito-urinary medicine clinic if discharge present.
Torsion (twisting) of the testis Sudden onset of disabling, excruciating pain in one testicle which is very painful to touch, and feels hard and high in scrotum. Nausea common. No fever.	See GP urgently or go straight to casualty. Requires operation within four hours of the start of the pain.
Epididymal cyst Firm swelling at end of one testicle, not usually painful to touch. Mild, dull and dragging pain; very gradual onset and may have been present for weeks or longer. Otherwise well.	See GP as soon as possible.
Stone in the ureter (calculus) Sudden, severe pain from one side of back, down through groin and into testicle (referred pain). Pain comes and goes in waves. Blood in urine possible; no fever.	See GP as soon as possible. Sieve urine with tea strainer to catch stones; retain them to show your GP.

Blood in the urine

Blood in the urine always needs to be investigated. It can sometimes be invisible to the eye and may be detected by a routine dipstick test at a medical checkup, or on microscopic examination. Invisible blood in the urine is usually a sign of an underlying problem.

OCCASIONAL CAUSES: jogging and hard exercise; cancer of the kidney; chronic interstitial cystitis; anticoagulant drugs; inflammation of the kidney (eg glomerulonephritis).
RARE CAUSES: renal tuberculosis; polycystic kidney disease; blood diseases (eg haemophilia, sickle-cell disease, thrombocytopaenia; infective endocarditis (heart inflammation); schistosomiasis (tropical disease).

COMMON CAUSES	ACTION
Urinary tract infection Burning, stinging pain on passing urine; frequent passing of small amounts. May have low backache.	Antibiotics are needed: see your GP urgently.
Bladder tumour There may be visible red blood in the urine, and difficulty in emptying the bladder.	See GP as soon as possible; requires specialist referral.
Urinary stones (calculi) in kidney or ureter Excruciating pain on one side of the back, often travelling down to the groin and into the penis, scrotum or vagina.	Call for GP visit for pain relief. Drink plenty of fluids. Later investigation necessary.
Urethritis (inflammation of the urethra) Pus discharge from bladder opening (urethra); stinging, burning pain on passing urine. Underlying cause is often a sexually transmitted disease.	Attend genito-urinary medicine clinic; requires antibiotics and investigation.
Enlarged prostate gland or cancer of prostate Gradual onset of difficulty in starting urination; slow urinary stream, and dribbling afterwards.	See GP non-urgently for examination and further investigation.

Incontinence, urinary

This is the involuntary passage of urine, largely a problem for women. It causes misery through its effect on people's personal hygiene, sexual relationships and ability to go out and about. It is estimated that urinary incontinence affects more than 30 per cent of women of all ages; over 50 per cent of incontinent women never seek help or do so only after many years of misery.

OCCASIONAL CAUSES: excessive urination (polyuria, see page 61); chronic urinary tract infection; interstitial cystitis; bladder stone; surgery or radiotherapy on abdomen and/or pelvis; abnormal opening (fistula), due to surgery or cancer.
RARE CAUSES: pelvic fracture; congenital abnormalities; nerve damage due to diabetes, syphilis, multiple sclerosis.

COMMON CAUSES	ACTION
Stress incontinence Leakage of small amounts of urine on coughing, straining or lifting. Perhaps caused by sphincter and/or pelvic floor damage through childbirth (often with prolapses).	See GP as soon as possible, or attend a local incontinence clinic.
Surgery to remove prostate gland (prostatectomy) Incontinence after a prostatectomy is usually only temporary.	Seek advice from your GP or hospital team as appropriate.
Urinary tract infections, especially cystitis Low, deep, dull, constant pain; often also felt in the back or higher on one side. Urgent desire to pass urine, but only small quantities are passed. Burning pain on passing urine, which may smell offensive and/or be bloodstained. Fever and feeling unwell.	See GP urgently.
Unstable bladder muscle This may follow, for example, a stroke, dementia or Parkinson's disease. It often disturbs sleep. The urge to pass urine may be so powerful that a toilet is not reached in time.	Restrict fluid intake in evenings. See GP as soon as possible.
Chronic outflow obstruction Gradual slowing of flow, difficulty starting urination, dribbling on stopping. Obstruction may be caused by enlargement of the prostate, narrowing of the urethra or bladder neck.	See GP as soon as possible.

Urination, excessive

Passing increased amounts of urine is nearly always associated with increased thirst.
The medical name is polyuria. (For more frequent passing of normal quantities of urine, see Urinary frequency below. For Urinary retention, see page 62.)

OCCASIONAL CAUSES: relief of chronic urinary obstruction; drugs (eg demeclocycline, lithium carbonate, amphotericin B, gentamicin); low potassium in blood (hypokalaemia); diabetes insipidus; Cushing's syndrome; sickle-cell anaemia; early chronic pyelonephritis (kidney inflammation).
RARE CAUSES: compulsive water-drinking (psychogenic polydipsia).

COMMON CAUSES	ACTION
Diabetes mellitus Continuous, marked thirst. Feeling tired and unwell; weight loss. Abdominal pain and/or vomiting if blood sugar levels very high.	See GP as soon as possible, urgently if you feel unwell. Take fresh urine sample for sugar testing.
Diuretic treatment Symptom usually worse for first few hours after taking treatment. Thirst not usually a problem.	See GP non-urgently if symptom causing major problems.
Excess alcohol intake The need to urinate is increased for several hours during and after excess drinking of alcohol. Dry mouth, hangover later.	Drink plenty of water to replace fluid lost. Avoid alcoholic bingeing.
Chronic kidney failure Often there are no symptoms; possible loss of appetite and weight.	See GP as soon as possible.
High calcium level in blood (hypercalcaemia) May result from, for example, osteoporosis treatment, cancer spread to bones, Paget's disease or hyperparathyroidism. Thirst is continuous. Generally unwell, with muscle cramps or spasms. Possible abdominal pain and vomiting.	See GP urgently or call for a home visit if you are too ill to travel.

Urinary frequency

Urinary frequency is the frequent passing of urine in usually small amounts. If large amounts of urine are passed frequently, this is excessive urination, covered above. (For Urinary retention, see page 62.)

OCCASIONAL CAUSES: inflamed prostate (prostatitis); non-infective interstitial cystitis; stone in the ureter; urethritis (inflammation of the urethra); pyelonephritis (kidney inflammation); thickening and narrowing of the bladder neck (bladder neck hypertrophy); tumour or swelling within the pelvis; habit.
RARE CAUSES: secondary to pelvic inflammation (eg pelvic infection, appendicitis, diverticulitis, adjacent tumour); benign or malignant bladder tumour.

COMMON CAUSES	ACTION
Infective cystitis (bladder infection) Dull, constant pain in stomach, back or kidney area on one side. Urgent desire to pass urine, but little passed, with burning pain. Urine may smell bad and/or be bloodstained.	See GP urgently for assessment.
Bladder stone (calculus) Urinary frequency preceded at some point by excruciating pain that may begin on one side of the abdomen or back. Blood often seen in urine. Frequency intermittent, eased by lying down. Passing urine may be painful or slow.	See GP as soon as possible.
Unstable bladder muscle This may follow, for example, a stroke, dementia, Parkinson's disease. Often disturbs sleep. Urge to pass urine may be so powerful that a toilet is not reached in time.	Restrict fluid intake in evenings. See GP as soon as possible.
Chronic outflow obstruction Gradual slowing of flow, difficulty in starting urination and dribbling on stopping. May be caused by, for example, enlarged prostate or narrowing of bladder neck or urethra.	See GP as soon as possible.
Anxiety Usually long-term, worse with stress and cold weather; fast, racing heartbeat, palpitations, nervous state. Sweaty skin, shaky hands; often breathlessness and pins and needles.	Consider ways to reduce life stress. See GP as soon as possible.

Many other symptoms require medical attention. This quick reference guide helps you to identify some of the most important. The heading indicates what action to take and how urgently to take it.

Emergency: get immediate medical advice/dial 999

Blood in vomit
If blood has been in the stomach for several hours, the vomit looks dark, like coffee grounds. Blood from the stomach passing through the gut turns the faeces jet black and tarry; it is very offensive to smell. Bleeding into the stomach can suddenly get worse. If coughing up blood, see page 24.

Breathing difficulty, sudden and severe in children (stridor)
Anxiety increases the problem, so remain outwardly calm and try to comfort the child while arranging help. In cases of acute airways obstruction by an inhaled foreign body, hold infants upside down and thump the back with the flat of the hand; perform the Heimlich manoeuvre in children too heavy to lift easily (see FIRST AID). Congenital laryngeal paralysis, which is usually detected immediately after birth in hospitals, accounts for one in four infants with stridor; in these cases follow hospital advice. (For shortness of breath in adults, see Breathlessness, chronic and Breathlessness, sudden, both page 22).

Confusion, sudden and severe
Any sudden, severe disorientation or delirium requires urgent hospital investigation to find the cause. For long term (chronic) confusion, see Memory loss, page 18.

Hallucinations
These are defined as the perception of something not actually there. Hallucinations require urgent medical attention as they may indicate medical conditions such as drug overdose, alcohol withdrawal, acute schizophrenia and other acute psychiatric conditions.

Loss of vision, sudden
It is sensible to go straight to casualty if vision is lost suddenly, especially if the eye is painful (see page 39). For gradual loss of vision, see page 63.

Urinary retention
The severe pain of an enlarged bladder needs urgent relief throught the passing of a tube (catheter) into the bladder, usually through the opening of the urinary tube (urethra). In general, it is quickest and best to attend a casualty department for treatment. For excessive or frequent urination, see page 61.

Urgent but not an emergency: get GP appointment or advice within 24 hours

Ear discharge
This is most commonly caused by an infection requiring antibiotic treatment. For earache, see page 38.

Facial pain
This is often caused by dental problems, including abscesses and jaw joint dysfunction (joint pain, cracking sound on movement). Visit a dentist before seeing a GP.

Facial swelling
See GP urgently or go to casualty if you suspect an allergy (sudden onset); dial 999 if there is difficulty in breathing, or swelling inside the mouth. For swelling, pain and bruising following a blow to the head, go to casualty for X-rays; don't take food or drink until seen. For a dental abscess, see a dentist urgently.

Facial ulcers and blisters
In children, rapidly developing and spreading golden-crusted sores, often around the mouth, may be impetigo. In older people, blisters may indicate shingles (herpes zoster). Both are contagious. For other rashes, blisters and pus spots, see pages 27 to 33.

Fever, prolonged
Seek help for fever of more than three or four days. Mention any recent foreign travel.

Jaundice
Yellow discoloration of the skin and the whites of the eyes caused by deposits of bile pigments. Indicates excessive breakdown of blood cells, a failure of the liver to work properly, or a blockage of the bile ducts.

Jaw, painful and/or swelling
Go to a casualty department for a suspected fracture (inability to open the mouth much). Visit a dentist urgently for dental causes such as: abscess or cyst (severe dull ache and swelling; swollen neck glands and fever); jaw joint dysfunction (pain and possible cracking sound on movement); unerupted teeth; gum swelling.

Loss of consciousness
See GP urgently if also fast or irregular heartbeats and shortness of breath; dial 999 if symptoms are jerkiness of limbs and grunting breathing; this may be epilepsy. For falls with no loss of consciousness, see page 63.

Important but not urgent: get next available GP appointment

Abnormal eating
Although difficult to persuade the person to visit a doctor, it is important to do so before the problem gets out of hand. (See also Weight gain and Weight loss, page 21.)

Abnormal gait in adults
Make an urgent GP appointment or ask for a home visit if symptoms include disabling vertigo, nausea and vomiting; it may be labyrinthitis, a viral infection. For limping in a child, see page 36.

Excessive body hair
This affects both men and women, but usually refers to excess body hair in a male distribution on a woman (that is, on the face, lower abdomen and upper thighs). There is usually no particular cause. See a GP if it has appeared suddenly; otherwise, see a cosmetician for treatment.

Falls with no loss of consciousness
Such falls are not usually serious, although if a sudden fall accompanies any acute illness, such as a stroke, see GP urgently or ask for home visit. These can be caused by, for example, low blood pressure, poor blood supply to the brain or medication.

Flushing lasting for several minutes
Emotional flushing that lasts seconds, and affects only the face, is normal. If severe or unusually frequent, it can be a sign of an underlying problem; seek a GP's advice.

Faecal incontinence
Most causes are non-urgent: severe haemorrhoids (piles), rectal prolapse, severe constipation or childbirth. Urgent medical attention is required for sudden onset of faecal incontinence with severe back pain and numbness in the back of the thighs; this could indicate a centrally prolapsed lumbar disc. For rectal bleeding and discharge, see pages 49 and 50. For urinary incontinence, see page 60.

Loss of vision, gradual
Emergency or urgent treatment is not needed for most causes, for example, cataracts or long-term damage from diabetes or high blood pressure. But persistent early-morning headaches with double vision may indicate a serious cause. See GP urgently if there is gradual loss of part of the field of vision: this may be creeping inferior retinal detachment, and urgent laser treatment referral may be needed. For sudden loss of vision, see page 62. For painful eyes, see page 39.

Nipple discharge
In general, although infection needs to be dealt with quickly, most causes, such as pregnancy or a reaction to certain drugs, do not need urgent medical attention. An areolar abscess (pus discharge, sometimes bloodstained, from one breast; underlying tissue hot and excruciatingly painful to touch), however, may require immediate surgery, so urgent GP assessment is required. For breast pain and lumps, see page 51.

Nose, blocked
Seek advice from a GP for a blocked nose that is not associated with a simple cold and lasts four weeks or more. For nosebleeds, see page 42.

Puberty, delayed
Delayed puberty is a failure to develop adult sexual characteristics by age 15 in boys, and 14 in girls (or failure to start periods by age 16). Have it investigated by your GP.

Vaginal bleeding, irregular
Menstrual periods are normal vaginal bleeding in women of reproductive age. Any bleeding outside of periods, before puberty or after the menopause is not normal and should be discussed with a GP. If irregular bleeding is associated with discoloured vaginal discharge and pelvic pain, get an urgent GP appointment or go to a genito-urinary medicine clinic; this may be cervicitis (inflammation of the cervix) or a pelvic infection, which need antibiotics. See also Pelvic pain, severe and sudden, page 53.

Vertigo
This symptom manifests itself in the illusion of movement, either of the head or the surroundings; nausea is often present as well. Its causes are quite different from those of dizziness (see Lightheadedness, page 17), and although it is not life-threatening, its effects can be disabling and distressing. In cases of severe vertigo where travel is impossible, ask for a home visit. See GP urgently if vertigo appears suddenly and is severe and continuous, as the cause may be viral (for example, a cold or tinnitus). Otitis media (middle ear infection that appears suddenly with severe pain, discharge and deafness on the same side, possible fever and tinnitus) also needs urgent treatment.

Abdominal pain

The abdomen – the lower part of the trunk, running from the diaphragm to the pelvis – contains many of the body's vital organs, including the stomach, kidneys and liver. The abdominal cavity is enclosed at the front by layers of skin and fat and at the back by the spine and lower ribs. The organs in the abdomen are sealed within a smooth, thin membrane called the peritoneum. If this is broken, bacteria can enter the cavity and cause a serious infection (see **Peritonitis**).

TYPES OF ABDOMINAL PAIN

Abdominal pain may be short-lived or chronic (recurring)and felt in various areas. It can take many forms and may be described as griping, gnawing, boring, deep grinding, nagging, bloating, colicky, cramping and stabbing.

▼ Abdominal pain

The red areas show the abdominal regions where pain is most often felt. Sudden and sharp pain felt in any of these places is most likely to be digestion related. Medical advice should always be sought for pain that continues for more than 24 hours.

Oesophagus

Liver

Stomach

Gall bladder

Large intestine

Small intestine

Appendix

Colon

Rectum

Because the abdominal cavity contains various body organs and systems, there are many possible causes of abdominal pain. In addition, pain in other areas of the body can suggest a problem in the abdominal area. Pain in the liver, for example, may be felt in the right shoulder. This is known as referred pain.

DIAGNOSIS

To help with diagnosis a doctor may gently investigate tender areas with his or her fingers. He or she may also tap the abdomen; a dull rather than a resonant sound may suggest the presence of fluid or a growth. A stethoscope may be used to listen for abnormal bowel sounds; unusually loud sounds can indicate enteritis (inflammation of the small intestine) or minor digestive problems. The doctor will also take account of any other symptoms, such as swelling, diarrhoea, constipation, abnormal stools, urinary problems, wind, heartburn, vomiting, vaginal bleeding and heavy, painful periods (see also **Symptom sorter**).

CAUSES OF ABDOMINAL PAIN

Abdominal pain may be caused by food poisoning, which may also lead to diarrhoea, vomiting and constipation. Other causes include menstrual problems or pregnancy, **hiatus hernia**, stomach or duodenal **ulcer**, or other damage to the structure of the abdomen. In children, psychological factors, wind, **colic**, appendicitis or inflammation of the lymph glands around the intestines may be responsible. Otherwise, abdominal pain is generally the result of a disorder that affects one of the organs or systems that the abdomen contains.

SEE ALSO *Bladder and disorders; Bowel and disorders; Cancer; Digestive system; Gallbladder and disorders; Kidneys and disorders; Liver and disorders; Pancreas and disorders; Spleen and disorders; Stomach and disorders; Urinary system*

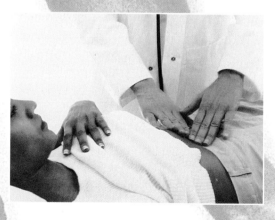

▲ Rebound pain

If pain intensifies when pressure is released, it can indicate appendicitis.

Abortion

An abortion is the expulsion or removal of an embryo or fetus from the uterus. A miscarriage is a naturally occurring abortion, known medically as spontaneous abortion. It may be caused by a number of factors, including abnormalities in the fetus or in the uterus, and genetic or hormonal disorders. Elective abortion is the deliberate termination of a pregnancy for medical or social reasons. Deliberate termination of a pregnancy has been legal in Britain, but not Northern Ireland, since 1967.

WHEN IS TERMINATION PERMITTED?

Where legal, termination can be performed at any time up to 24 weeks after conception if two doctors agree that continuing the pregnancy poses a serious risk to the physical or mental health of the woman or her family, or that the baby is likely to have a serious handicap.

HOW IS TERMINATION PERFORMED?

Three methods are used.
- Up to nine weeks after conception, the drug mifepristone is given to disrupt the pregnancy; a prostaglandin pessary is then inserted to activate uterine contractions and expel the fetus.
- Up to around 14 weeks, the contents of the uterus are removed by suction.
- After 14 weeks, either the fetus is removed surgically or prostaglandin is administered to induce contractions.

SEE ALSO *Miscarriage; Pregnancy, termination of*

Abscess

An abscess is a collection of pus produced when white blood cells flood into an area of the body, usually to destroy invading bacteria. Abscesses may occur internally – for example, in the teeth, liver, gut, lungs, brain or breast – and may result from conditions such as **appendicitis** or **peritonitis**. A **boil** is a small abscess that forms around a hair follicle in the skin.

SYMPTOMS
- A red, hot, painful swelling.
- Raised temperature and sweating.
- General feeling of illness and loss of appetite.
- Internal abscesses may produce pain or symptoms such as **diarrhoea** or a **cough**.

CAUSES
- Usually bacterial infection, but may be due to irritants entering the tissues.
- Infection is more likely if body defences are weak, as in people with **diabetes** or poor nutrition, or who are suffering from stress.
- Sometimes an abscess is caused by the spread of infection, as in brain abscesses that result from lung, middle ear or sinus infections.

TREATMENT
Small abscesses, such as boils, may be left untreated but larger ones will need treatment to drain the pus.

What you can do
For a small, localized abscess such as a boil:
- apply heat or a magnesium sulphate poultice to encourage the boil to come to a head;
- take **paracetamol** for pain;
- rest and eat healthily;
- keep flannels separate from those of other household members, and wash carefully before preparing food, to avoid spreading infection.

When to consult a doctor
See your doctor if:
- you develop a fever or **cellulitis**, or begin to feel unwell;
- an external abscess becomes larger than a simple boil, is painful or does not improve;
- the redness spreads to the surrounding skin without the boil coming to a head;
- the boils are recurrent or persistent, or the discharge is continual.

What a doctor may do
Depending on how advanced the abscess is, the doctor may:
- prescribe **antibiotics**;
- lance the abscess with a sterile needle to allow the pus to drain;
- arrange for you to be admitted to hospital for surgical drainage. Any cavity formed by the abscess will then need to be packed with dressing, to allow it to continue draining and healing. If the cavity is allowed to close up, the abscess may re-form. Swabs will identify any bacteria behind the infection, and you will be screened for undiagnosed diabetes.

Complementary therapies
These are generally no substitutes for the orthodox medical treatment of large abscesses, but complementary treatments may help first aid or prevention.
- **Homeopathy:** try Hepar sulph (Hep.) and Silicea (Sil.) to speed drainage; and Belladonna (Bell.) to cope with throbbing pain.
- **Naturopathy:** a wholefood diet may help to prevent recurrent boils.

COMPLICATIONS
- If an untreated abscess bursts, pus will leak onto the nearest surface. The drained pus from an internal abscess may then collect in a new cavity and form another abscess.
- Infection may spread from an abscess to cause **septicaemia** or may lead to a more extensive infection such as **osteomyelitis, meningitis, encephalitis** or **peritonitis**.
- A brain abscess may be fatal unless it is drained rapidly, or it may leave the person with **epilepsy**.

Accident prevention

More people are injured in their own homes than at work or on the street. Identifying potentially hazardous areas and taking a few inexpensive precautions can significantly reduce everyday risks.

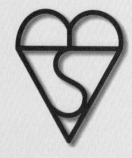

▲ **Mark of safety**
The British Standards Institution kitemark on a product indicates that prescribed safety standards have been met by the maker.

The most dangerous areas in and around the home are the kitchen, the living and dining areas, the stairs and the garden. Most accidents are caused by human error, but faulty appliances, mechanical defects, poor house-wiring and gas leaks are all potentially hazardous.

Every year, 2.7 million people in the UK attend hospital as a result of accidents in the home. One million of those are children, half of whom are under five years old. Almost four thousand people die following accidents in the home each year, compared with about 3600 road deaths.

Even minor injury brings unnecessary pain, so it makes sense to ensure that your home is as safe as it possibly can be. Although it is not possible to make a home totally accident-proof, there are various products on the market that will make your home a safer place to be.

■ Portable residual current devices (RCDs) protect against danger from faults in electrically powered household and garden tools. Tools should be plugged into an RCD before use; the device breaks the circuit in the event of a fault.

■ Ten-year sealed-cell smoke alarms bypass the need for annual battery replacement. Vibrating alarms and alarms with strobe lights are available for people with poor hearing or eyesight.

■ Curly flexes for kettles and other similar appliances eliminate trailing cords, which can get caught up in crockery and cause accidents.

Child safety tips

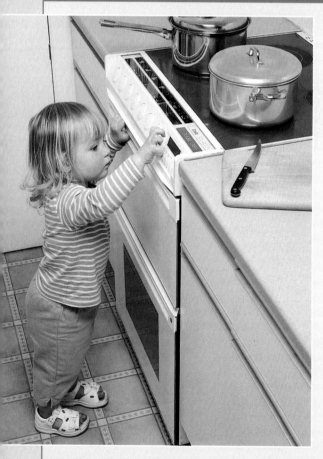

Always supervise children at play. Up until about the age of 12, children are unable to recognize and understand danger fully. Curiosity, a spirit of adventure and a tendency to show off expose them to risk at every turn.

■ Use child-resistant gadgets where available: safety gates, fireguards, safety plugs and door latches.

■ Install window-opening restrictors.

■ Ensure that hot liquids are kept well away from children: a scald caused by a spillage of hot tea can scar a child for life.

■ When filling a bath for a child, start by running the cold water, then top it up with hot water, to avoid scalding.

■ Never leave a baby alone when he or she is feeding.

◀ **Danger in the kitchen**
For children, the kitchen is a dangerous place. Keep pan handles out of reach and be aware of danger areas within your child's reach – many surfaces remain hot even when the power is off.

■ Don't let children run around when they are carrying scissors, knives or pencils.

■ Take care over how you store sharp objects – for example, don't load knives in a dishwasher with the blades sticking upwards.

■ Keep all medicines out of reach, preferably in a locked cabinet.

■ Never decant medicines or household cleaners into other containers.

■ Buy toys that are appropriate for a child's age.

■ Shallow water is dangerous both inside and outside the house. Never leave a child alone in the bath. In an average year, 11 under-fives drown in garden ponds. Cover or fence off your garden pond – or, better still, fill it in. Take extra care when you take your child to visit unfamiliar gardens with ponds or pools.

Ensure that all your gas appliances are installed, repaired and given an annual check by a company that is registered with the Council for Registered Gas Installers (CORGI). Blocked flues can cause carbon monoxide poisoning.

People move and react more slowly as they grow older, and take longer to get out of danger's way. Poor eyesight, hearing and balance can make even the most familiar environment risky. Fitting an alarm that alerts a relative, neighbour or professional helper is a good idea.

Take care when working with garden tools, and use a residual current device (RCD), or circuit breaker, with all electric tools. Don't forget that electric mower blades rotate for some time after the power has been turned off. Store sharp tools in a locked cupboard and use protective gloves for gardening. If hiring power tools, use a reputable hire shop, ask for safety advice and a demonstration. Maintain garden paths and driveways. Keep surfaces level and free from moss and leaves.

Candles create a pleasant atmosphere, but also pose a fire risk. Read the instructions for use and place candles in stable containers away from curtains. Never leave candles unattended and always extinguish them carefully.

Make sure that any necessary medicine is taken in the right doses and at the correct times. Keep medicines out of reach of children, preferably in a locked cabinet.

Have your wiring checked by a professional. Never put a portable electrical device in a bathroom.

Check that upholstery conforms to the latest fire safety regulations, available from your local fire brigade.

If you smoke, use an ashtray. Never smoke in bed, in the garage or near a car when the engine is running.

Install a phone line and a panic alarm system; carry a mobile phone for emergency contact.

In the garage or driveway, ensure that the car is locked and the handbrake is on. Never leave the ignition key in place. Do not start the engine with the garage door shut. Check daily for oil and other leaks. Store petrol away from the garage in a locked shed.

Don't overload power points with multiway adaptors. Install more power points instead. Turn off the TV at night and pull out the plug.

To prevent falls, secure carpet edges with metal strips and remove loose mats – especially on shiny floors. Pick up all objects that could be tripped over. Install good lighting.

Never leave an open fire unguarded. If you have young children, install a fixed-surround fireguard. Have the chimney swept annually. Install smoke alarms and check them regularly; change the batteries each year unless you are using ten-year sealed-cell models.

Keep a fire blanket in the kitchen to smother small fires. In the case of a major fire, leave the house at once, and call the fire brigade. Know your escape routes and practise using them.

CONTACT **Local council** Ask for the home safety officer or environmental health officer **The Royal Society for the Prevention of Accidents (RoSPA)** (0121) 248 2000 **Child Accident Prevention Trust (CAPT)** (020) 7608 3828 (www.capt.org.uk) **The Council for Registered Gas Installers (CORGI)** (01256) 372200

ACE inhibitors

ACE inhibitors (angiotensin-converting enzyme inhibitors) are drugs used to treat hypertension and **heart failure**, and to protect the kidneys of diabetics. ACE inhibitors such as captopril and enalapril maleate block the action of an enzyme in the blood that produces the hormone angiotensin II which narrows the blood vessels. Inhibiting this action causes a widening of the vessels, a fall in blood pressure and a reduced workload for the heart. They are often taken with **diuretics**. Side effects of ACE inhibitors may include a persistent dry cough, nausea and vomiting, itching, a rash and taste changes.

ADVICE ON USAGE

A low dose at bedtime avoids lightheadedness and giddiness. Avoid taking non-steroidal anti-inflammatory drugs (NSAIDs) such as aspirin in addition to ACE inhibitors, since there is a risk of kidney damage, and salt substitutes containing potassium. ACE inhibitors should not be used in pregnancy, so tell your doctor if you are pregnant or planning to conceive.

SEE ALSO **Blood pressure and problems; Drugs, medicinal**

Acetone

Acetone is one of three biochemical compounds known as ketones, produced when fats are used by the body as fuel. Extreme diets, and certain diabetic conditions cause high levels of ketones in the blood. Ketoacidosis occurs when acetone and related ketones reach a certain level; it may lead to a hyperglycaemic coma.

SEE ALSO **Acidosis; Diabetes; Hyperglycaemia**

Achalasia

Achalasia is a rare condition in which the muscles of the oesophagus lose their efficiency. As a result, the muscle guarding the stomach's opening does not relax to allow food through. The cause may be nerve damage, a tumour or a parasitic infection. Symptoms include difficulty with swallowing, chest pain and a cough. To treat achalasia, the standard treatment involves undergoing keyhole surgery.

SEE ALSO **Oesophagus and disorders**

Achilles tendon rupture

The achilles is a thick, strong tendon (a cord made up of bundles of collagen fibres) behind the ankle that anchors the calf muscles to the heel bone. Rupture can occur during energetic sport, particularly if the calf muscles have not been warmed up, and usually requires surgery.

SEE ALSO **Tendons and disorders**

Achondroplasia

Achondroplasia is one of a number of bone conditions causing short stature (once called dwarfism). The upper arms and thighs are most affected, resulting in an average height for an achondroplasic woman of 1.23m (4ft) and for a man of 1.32m (4ft 4in). People affected have a normal lifespan and intelligence. It is a rare, inherited condition, affecting some 25–30 babies born in the UK each year.

SEE ALSO **Genetics and genetic disorders**

Acid regurgitation

Also known as **heartburn**, acid regurgitation is a backflow of acid from the stomach into the oesophagus that occurs when the muscle at the entry point of the stomach is weak or relaxes inappropriately. Fatty and fried foods, smoking cigarettes and alcohol abuse are all causes of acid regurgitation, but the problem may also be associated with pregnancy or a **hiatus hernia**.

SEE ALSO **Diet; Indigestion; Oesophagus and disorders**

Acidosis

Acidosis is a condition in which too much acid accumulates in the blood and body fluids. There are various kinds. One of these is ketoacidosis, caused by the body's breaking down muscle and fat and producing ketones. It results from uncontrolled diabetes, alcoholism or extreme diets such as high-protein diets.

SEE ALSO **Alkalosis**

Acne rosacea

Acne rosacea, commonly called rosacea, is an inflammatory skin condition that affects around one per cent of the UK population. The majority of sufferers are fair-skinned women aged 30–50.

The causes of rosacea are unknown but they are thought to include abnormal sensitivity of blood capillaries and infection of sebaceous (oil) glands with a skin mite, *Demodex folliculorum*. Rosacea tends to recur over a five- to ten-year period, after which it may clear up completely.

SYMPTOMS

Acne rosacea is evident in several ways:
- Flushing, especially after drinking alcohol, eating spicy food, consuming hot drinks or entering a warm room.
- Small pimples.
- Fine, dilated skin capillaries (telangiectasia).
- Left untreated, the skin remains permanently red with small, pus-filled blisters called pustules.

TREATMENT

Seek medical advice. Your doctor may prescribe oral **antibiotics** or metronidazole gel, or refer you to a dermatologist.

Avoid stress, hot liquids, spicy foods, alcohol, vigorous exercise and exposure to sunlight. Avoiding tea, chocolate, cheese, yeast extract, eggs, citrus fruits and wheat may help.

Complementary therapies

- Rosacea may respond to vitamin B complex.
- Natural antiparasitic agents such as tea tree oil applied to the skin may be effective.
- Aloe vera gel helps to reduce inflammation.

CONTACT **Acne Support Group** PO Box 9, Newquay, Cornwall TR9 6WG
0870 870 2263
SEE ALSO *Rosacea*

Acne vulgaris

Acne vulgaris is an inflammatory skin disease. It affects the sebaceous (oil) glands within the hair follicles on the face, outer ear canal, back, chest and groin. In severe cases, acne may spread as far as the legs. The condition usually starts at puberty and peaks at 17–21.

Four out of five teenagers suffer from acne, which can be an embarrassing condition. One per cent of men and five per cent of women in the UK have problems after the age of 40.

SYMPTOMS

- Greasy skin.
- Spots and pimples on the face, shoulders, back or chest.
- In severe cases, inflamed cysts deep in the skin.

CAUSES

Acne is caused by increased activity of the skin's sebaceous glands influenced by sex hormones called androgens. Blockage of the duct leading from the gland to the skin traps secretions inside to form blackheads. Increased numbers of bacteria on the skin occur, and can become trapped inside the ducts. Bacterial enzymes break down skin oil to trigger inflammation.

Boys are more prone to acne than girls because they have higher androgen levels, but many girls also suffer, usually in the week before their menstrual period starts.

TREATMENT

Seek help early. Mild acne can respond well to over-the-counter preparations; severe acne needs prescription drugs. Many women find that the contraceptive pill is effective. With continuous treatment, nine out of ten people show 80 per cent improvement within six months.

Complementary therapies

Tea tree oil products are often effective.

COMPLICATIONS

Severe acne can leave scars; plastic surgery and other cosmetic treatments may help.

CONTACT **Acne Support Group** PO Box 9, Newquay, Cornwall TR9 6WG
0870 870 2263

Acoustic neuroma

An acoustic neuroma is a tumour in the hearing nerve. Although rare, it accounts for five per cent of all tumours within the skull. The early symptoms, **dizziness** and tinnitus, do not in themselves suggest serious disease, but seek medical advice if deafness occurs, especially if it is only in one ear. Diagnosis is by hearing tests and a **magnetic resonance imaging** (MRI) scan.
SEE ALSO *Ear and problems*

Acrocyanosis

Acrocyanosis makes the hands and feet go cold and blue. Swelling or sweating may also occur, but there is no pain. The condition mainly affects women. The cause is unknown, but cold makes it worse. Sympathectomy (keyhole surgery or injection that severs the nerves which control the arterioles) may relieve symptoms.

Acromegaly

Acromegaly is a chronic metabolic disorder in which too much growth hormone is produced by the **pituitary gland**. The bones of the face, jaw, hands, feet and skull enlarge. It is usually a result of a benign tumour of the pituitary.

Acroparaesthesia

An intense tingling or pricking in the fingers or toes is known as acroparaesthesia. The usual cause is restricted blood supply to the nerves due to resting heavily on a limb during sleep or by a long period of inactivity. Repeated bouts may indicate nerve inflammation or damage.

Acupressure

Acupressure forms part of the system of traditional Chinese medicine that dates back more than 2000 years. Like **acupuncture**, it is based on the principle that *qi*, or *chi*, meaning 'life force', flows constantly through the body. Any overactivity, blockage or slowing down of *qi* can result in illness. Pressure on certain points (acupoints) on the 12 main energy channels in the body, known as meridians, is thought to regulate the flow of the body's energy, allowing balance to be restored and stimulating the body to heal itself.

The practitioner uses thumb and fingertip pressure to work the appropriate acupoints, rather than the fine needles that are used for the same purpose in acupuncture.

HOW IT CAN HELP

Acupressure is a non-invasive alternative to acupuncture that you can do at home. Acupuncturists may offer it to people who dislike the idea of needles. It is used to treat:
- pain, including chronic back pain, arthritic pain, headaches and migraine;
- nausea;
- gynaecological problems;
- stress and stress-related conditions.

WHAT'S INVOLVED

At your first appointment the practitioner will ask you for a full medical and lifestyle history, and will also take your pulse and inspect your tongue to aid diagnosis.

As well as working on the appropriate acupoints, the practitioner may also show you how to use acupressure as a self-help therapy. The first session will probably last at least an hour; subsequent sessions are likely to take 30–45 minutes.

CONTACT **The British Acupuncture Council** 63 Jeddo Road, London W12 9HQ (020) 8735 0400
Institute for Complementary Medicine PO Box 194, London SE16 7QZ (020) 7237 5165

Acupuncture

Practised in China for more than 2000 years, acupuncture is a form of complementary therapy now offered in NHS pain clinics and recommended by an increasing number of orthodox doctors. It is based on the belief that illness or disease is caused by blockages or imbalances in *qi*, or *chi*, the 'life force' that flows through the body.

Acupuncturists insert fine needles into certain points (called acupoints) on the body's energy channels (meridians) to promote the flow of *qi* and, ultimately, to bring the body back to its natural state of equilibrium. Western scientists have detected what may be evidence for the existence of *qi*. According to the Institute of Electrical and Electronics Engineers, the skin above the acupoints has a lower electrical resistance than the surrounding skin.

HOW IT CAN HELP

The effectiveness of acupuncture in the treatment of digestive problems, respiratory disease, pain, neurological disorders, nausea and a range of gynaecological ailments – from premenstrual syndrome to infertility and the menopause – has been officially acknowledged by the World Health Organization. Acupuncture is also often used to treat stress and stress-related conditions.

THE ORTHODOX VIEW

The traditional view among conventional doctors is that acupuncture works by:
- blocking the body's pain receptors (so that, even though pain signals are still being sent out, the person does not register them);
- stimulating the nervous system;
- encouraging the production of **endorphins**, hormone-like chemicals that enhance mood and are natural painkillers;
- promoting circulation of the blood.

FINDING A PRACTITIONER

Ask your GP for a referral to an NHS pain clinic, or contact The British Acupuncture Council or The British Medical Acupuncture Society for details of qualified practitioners in your area.

Before arranging treatment, check how long your chosen practitioner trained for, especially if he or she is an orthodox doctor. Some doctors

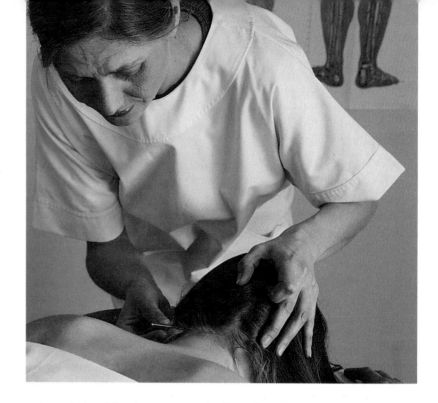

▲ **Painless therapy**
The acupuncturist may gently move the needle by rotating or vibrating it – many people feel no more than a slight tingling or numbness in the area.

Acupuncture is routinely used in China in place of the anaesthetic drugs that we rely on in the West. Beijing's Gynaecological and Obstetric Hospital carries out around 7000 Caesareans each year – and 1000 of these are performed using acupuncture.

who belong to The British Medical Acupuncture Society are permitted to practise a certain level of acupuncture after a four-day introductory course; other doctors have undergone a three-year training programme. Many non-medical acupuncturists train for at least two or three years, some for five years or more.

WHAT'S INVOLVED

The acupuncturist will ask you in detail about your medical history and current symptoms, about any other treatments you are having, your emotional well-being, your lifestyle and your family's medical history. The acupuncturist will take your pulse and inspect your tongue to help with diagnosis.

After diagnosis, the practitioner will decide what size of needles to use, where to place them and how long to leave them in. Fine stainless-steel needles will then be inserted into the relevant acupoints – usually in a different part of the body from the one that has the problem. The insertion is swift and painless and the most that you should feel is a slight prick. Tell your practitioner if the needles become uncomfortable during treatment. The needles are left in place for 10–30 minutes before being gently and painlessly withdrawn. Your first session should last up to 1¼ hours and further sessions are likely to be 30–45 minutes long. You may prefer to rest after treatment.

The number of treatments you need depends upon the type of health problem you have. In some cases, one or two sessions may be enough to resolve the problem. In others, you may need several treatments at weekly intervals, but you should notice a steady improvement. Many people also have regular appointments as a preventive measure.

Possible side effects

■ Swelling and discomfort around the site of needle insertion.
■ Brief worsening of symptoms before they begin to subside.

■ If inserted incorrectly, the needles can cause bleeding and even nerve damage. However, this is extremely rare.

Other treatments

Acupuncture treatment may also involve other techniques.
■ Moxibustion – the warming of acupoints with aromatic smoke from a bundle of the dried herb known as moxa (mugwort).
■ Cupping – placing small, bulbous glass cups over acupoints to create a partial vacuum, which then draws blood and *qi* into the area.
■ Electro-acupuncture – connecting the needles to a very small electrical current to increase the stimulation of particular acupoints.
■ **Acupressure** – stimulating the acupoints with finger pressure instead of needles.

HEALTH AND SAFETY

Sterilization of the needles used in acupuncture is crucial to prevent the transmission of infections such as HIV and viral hepatitis. Most acupuncturists use a new packet of needles for each patient. But needles are sometimes sterilized on site in a sterilizing machine known as an autoclave, or sent to a local hospital for sterilizing before being reused.

SEE ALSO ***Chinese herbal medicine***

CONTACT **The British Medical Acupuncture Society**
BMAS House, 3 Winnington Court, Northwich, Cheshire CW8 1AQ (01606) 786782 **The British Acupuncture Council** 63 Jeddo Road, London W12 9HQ (020) 8735 0400

Warning

If you have been fitted with a cardiac pacemaker, you should not undergo electro-acupuncture treatment.

Factfile

How acupuncture meridians are used

Many of the 20 meridians are named after the organs they serve.

Points on the channels can be used to treat problems in these organs – and in other parts of the body, too. For example, gall bladder points are used to ease hip joints or relieve migraines. Treatments often involve more than one meridian: kidney and lung points are used in combination to treat asthma.

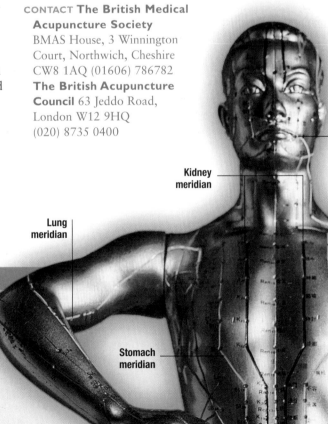

Large intestine meridian

Kidney meridian

Lung meridian

Stomach meridian

Liver meridian

Spleen meridian

Gall bladder meridian

Addictions

People with addictions often lose control of their lives. The most common addictions are to alcohol or drugs, but many different substances and activities can cause a dependency strong enough to dominate behaviour.

The term addiction usually implies a physical dependence on a substance. When a person has a physical addiction, abstaining from the addictive substance induces unpleasant withdrawal symptoms. This may occur with alcohol and drugs such as heroin, morphine and cocaine.

With psychological dependence there are no physical withdrawal symptoms, yet users come to rely on a substance or activity for a continued sense of well-being. This type of dependence can stem from the use of, for example, cannabis, amphetamines and tobacco. The word 'addiction' is also sometimes applied to excessive gambling, shopping, exercise, computer games, surfing the Internet or even promiscuous sex.

Both psychological and physical addictions can overpower people's capacity to make choices in their own best interests and may lead them into patterns of damaging behaviour.

THE HEALTH RISKS

Addictions carry a number of physical dangers as well as leading to personality changes.

■ Injecting drug users are vulnerable to infections such as **hepatitis** and **HIV**, which can be contracted through the use of infected injecting equipment.

■ Prolonged alcohol abuse is associated with a wide range of health risks including damage to the liver and nervous system, serious immune deficiency and an increased susceptibility to infections.

■ Tolerance of a particular substance may lead to a need for increasing doses to gain the same effect.

■ Drug users may be susceptible to death through overdose or physical reaction. For example, even occasional use of the drug Ecstasy carries the risk of death through dehydration and overheating.

THE ADDICTIVE PERSONALITY

Only a small proportion of people who use a drug become dependent on it. Whether or not someone becomes addicted to a substance depends on the person and the circumstances. For instance, many people treated medically with opiate **analgesic drugs** – painkillers that include diamorphine – do not become dependent on them, yet these are prime drugs of illegal use and subsequent addiction.

Some authorities believe that the personalities of certain people make them more vulnerable than others to developing an addiction, and that traits such as anxiety and impulsiveness may stem from the same gene patterns as those underlying addiction (see **Genetics and genetic disorders**).

Certain personality traits, such as sensation-seeking, are believed to lead some people into experimenting with, and using, social drugs. Certain 'pleasure chemicals' are released in the brain during activities such as eating and sexual activity, by sugar, gambling and risk-taking, and by some recreational drugs. It has been claimed that genes that determine the release of these 'pleasure chemicals' are deficient in some people and so they need a regular 'fix' from an outside source to feel good. However, most authorities think this is only one of many factors involved. Social environment, family background and availability of drugs may also be important.

Some experts believe that continued use of drugs or alcohol causes changes in the brain that increase the risk of addiction; it also leaves an imprint in the brain even after substance abuse has ceased – an 'addiction memory' – that can cause relapse at times of stress.

Signs of addiction

If you find unfamiliar substances, equipment or tablets lying around in your home, it may be that someone living with you is experimenting with illegal drugs. This may or may not indicate an addiction problem. Other signs of drug abuse and possible addiction can include:

■ poor performance at work;

■ difficulties in relationships;

■ financial problems;

■ lying and secretiveness about activities and acquaintances;

■ stealing;

■ in a teenager, a sudden worsening of performance at school or college, and a lack of concern about it; regularly coming home incoherent or 'spaced out'.

HOW TO BEAT ADDICTION

Start beating addiction by acknowledging your problem and the effects it is having on your life. Look for support from others in similar situations – people outside your immediate group of family and friends. You may need to seek professional help; few people can tackle addiction without it.

HELPING AN ADDICT

If a close friend or family member develops an addiction, there are several things you can do to help. Offering sympathy and support can be invaluable in helping someone to tackle the problem, but do not bail the person out of difficulties caused by addiction. This is usually counterproductive and may postpone the addict's recognition of the problem, or prolong the recovery period.

It is important to recognize that you are not in a position to end someone's addiction: the person needs professional help. Seek support through stress management, counselling or couple/family therapy, but do not expect this to change the problem or to improve your relationship with the addict.

SEE ALSO *Detoxification; Relaxation techniques; Smoking and problems; Solvent abuse*

CONTACT **Drinkline** 0800 917 8282 – free-phone counselling, support, advice and information on alcohol-related problems; 7am–11pm Mon–Fri; 24 hours over weekend **Frank** 0800 776600 (www.talktofrank.com) Government scheme with 24-hour freephone advice and information on drugs and solvents **Quitline** 0800 002200 – freephone for people wanting to give up smoking, 9am–9pm daily **Adfam** (020) 7928 8898 – working with the families and friends of drug users (www.adfam.org.uk)

Addison's disease

Addison's disease is a rare condition caused by a hormone deficiency. The deficiency can be caused either by disease of the **adrenal glands**, or the failure of the **pituitary glands** to produce enough adrenocorticotropic hormone (ACTH). Symptoms include increasing weakness and tiredness leading to complete exhaustion. The condition may occur temporarily when someone stops taking glucocorticoids, prescribed for illnesses such as rheumatoid arthritis and asthma.

Additives, food

Food additives are chemicals added during the processing of food. They are used to help to preserve foods, to assist in the manufacturing process, or to improve a food's taste, texture or appearance. Additives are also used in some **nutritional supplements** and medicines.

Many additives are naturally occurring substances, but this doesn't necessarily mean that they are harmless. Some people are sensitive to certain additives. Preservatives containing sulphur, for example, may pose a hazard to asthma sufferers. Some colourings, such as tartrazine, have been linked anecdotally with hyperactivity in children. Labelling regulations require additives to appear in the ingredients list, either by name or by 'E' number (see decoder below).

Some foods are required by law to remain free of additives, or to contain a restricted number. These include: milk, cream and live or fermented milk products; bottled water; natural coffee; leaf tea; and dried pasta.

E-additives decoder

All additives are given 'E' numbers approved by the European Union. Broad classifications are:

E-ADDITIVES	TYPE
E100 to E1801	colourings
E200 to E285	preservatives
E300 to E321	antioxidants
E322 to E495	emulsifiers, thickeners and stabilizers
E420, E421, E953 to E967	sweeteners
E500 to E507, E524 to E529	acids and acidity regulators
E551 to E559	anti-caking agents
E620 to E635	flavour enhancers
E901 to E914	glazing agents
E920	flour treatment agent
E938 to E949	gases involved in packaging

Adenitis

Adenitis is an inflammation of a gland or group of glands. The term is usually used to refer to lymph glands, especially those in the neck, armpit and groin, which are the glands most commonly affected (see **Lymphatic system**). Painful swelling of the glands is often associated with fever and indicates that the body is working to overcome an infection.

Adenoids and problems

The adenoids are the mass of lymphatic tissue at the back of the nasal cavity. The **tonsils**, at the back of the mouth, consist of the same tissue. Both form part of the **lymphatic system**, a network of lymph nodes linked by lymphatic vessels – which defends the body from infection.

Some areas of lymph tissue, such as those in the adenoids and tonsils, are largest during childhood and shrink throughout life.

WHAT CAN GO WRONG

Recurrent infections may lead to adenoid and tonsil enlargement. Enlarged adenoids can block the Eustachian tube that drains the middle ear, resulting in a buildup of fluid known as **glue ear**. This interferes with sound transmission, causing temporary deafness; in young children, this affects hearing and language skills development. The adenoids may also obstruct nose to throat air flow, forcing the child to breathe through the mouth. If mouth breathing becomes persistent, the child may develop a nasal voice and a dull facial expression. Evidence suggests that long-term reduced oxygen can impair brain function.

Depending on the severity of the symptoms and the age of the patient, a doctor may recommend surgery to remove the adenoids and possibly the tonsils at the same time.

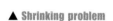

▲ **Shrinking problem**
The adenoids lie at the back of the nose close to where it joins the mouth. Small at birth, they start growing at around 18 months and reach maximum size at about the age of eight.

ADHD

ADHD (attention deficit hyperactivity disorder) is characterized by impulsiveness, inattention and overactivity. ADHD starts in childhood but it is a chronic condition and symptoms may persist into adolescence and adulthood.

In the UK, the disorder is formally diagnosed only when a child is persistently inattentive, impulsive and overactive from an early age, and the main features of the child's behaviour are evident in more than one setting – for example, both at home and in school. The syndrome is present in five per cent of schoolchildren in the UK, and is more common in boys. In the USA, the syndrome is diagnosed in three to six per cent of the school-aged population.

SYMPTOMS

A child with ADHD displays the following:
- impulsive and disruptive behaviour;
- impaired attention – inability to concentrate, short attention span;
- hyperactivity – inability to sit still, continual fidgeting and chattering, abundance of energy and need for only a little sleep.

TREATMENT

Although symptoms usually start in the preschool years, there is a wide range of normal behaviour in preschool children, so a definite diagnosis of ADHD may not be made until a child starts school. If you suspect that your child is suffering from ADHD, consult a doctor and talk to your child's teacher.

Before a diagnosis is made, the child will have a full mental health and behavioural assessment by the appropriate specialists.

Once a diagnosis is made, the child will be offered educational support and behavioural therapy such as social skills training.

In some children, symptoms are made more severe by particular foods or food additives, but no single food has been shown to affect all children with ADHD. You may wish to keep a food diary to check if any foods or additives make your child's problems worse.

School-aged children with severe ADHD or those for whom behavioural therapy does not work should be offered additional treatment in the form of a stimulant medication such as Ritalin (methylphenidate hydrochloride) or Dexedrine (dexamfetamine sulphate). These drugs are effective in relieving symptoms and may be taken for a number of years. There may be side effects, so drug use should be reviewed.

SEE ALSO *Behaviour problems in children*

CONTACT **Hyperactive Children's Support Group** 71 Whyke Lane, Chichester, West Sussex PO19 7PD; emergency helpline (01243) 551313 (www.hacsg.org.uk)
ADDISS PO Box 340, Edgware, Middlesex HA8 9HL (020) 8906 9068 (www.addiss.co.uk)

Adhesion

Adhesion is the term used to describe scar tissue that forms in the organs of the abdominal cavity as a result of abdominal surgery or an infection. Adhesions usually occur in the bowel and can cause kinking, resulting in pain and occasionally obstruction. Adhesions in the pelvic area can adversely affect a woman's fertility.

SEE ALSO *Scars*

Adolescence

Teenagers and their parents enter a challenging period in the transition between childhood and adulthood. Adolescents go through a range of new experiences, which make them consider how they see themselves.

Adolescence is the time when people first start to learn about the real world and to discover their place in it.

Every adolescent has to deal with not only the psychological effects of maturing physically but also the development of an independent adult identity. Body image – a crucial issue for all adolescents – is inextricably bound up with the physical changes that occur at **puberty**, as well as increasing sexual experimentation and teenagers' sense of their own attractiveness.

At the same time as adolescents are coming to terms with bodily development, their relationships with their parents and family are changing as peer group pressure and media influences encourage them to try out new ideas and new roles. The depth and extent of family love and care are severely put to the test when young people push to the limit the boundaries of what their parents consider acceptable. Although it can be a source of bitter conflict, this process is all about an adolescent's need to establish a separate identity while being reassured about the deep sense of security associated with the family group.

External factors such as examination pressures and career decisions compound the problems of becoming an adult. Developing sexuality carries with it concerns about **contraception** and **sexually transmitted diseases**, and adolescents must be prepared to face the temptations presented by alcohol, cigarettes and illegal drugs.

▼ Breaking free Adolescents respond well to increasing freedom in return for behaving responsibly.

LIVING WITH ADOLESCENTS
For parents, adolescence can be challenging, but you can reduce the potential for conflict by trying to adapt your own role to that of counsellor. Other survival strategies include the following:
- Stand firm over agreed and important rules (especially when it comes to safety).
- Seek to offer unconditional support and love.
- Accept that adolescents need to vent their frustrations – don't take outbursts personally.
- Don't probe or offer unsolicited advice.

ADOLESCENTS AND FOOD
A well-balanced diet is particularly important during adolescence, when some people double their body weight as a result of muscle development and increasing height (see **Diet**). Emotional stress and concern with self-image make some teenagers vulnerable to **anorexia nervosa** and other **eating disorders**.

COMMUNICATING WITH ADOLESCENTS
As a parent you may want to discuss with your adolescent children and their friends issues such as smoking, alcohol, drugs and sexual behaviour. The following guidelines may help.
- Try to be open, frank and available to talk.
- Listen to what your child has to say.
- Accept that you can guide but can't control.
- Boost adolescents' self-esteem – which is vital if they are to learn to say 'no' to others.
- Offer accurate factual information.
- Stress your concern for your child's well-being.
- Recognize that adolescents mature earlier today.
- Discuss relationships as well as sex.
- Try not to overreact.
- Don't smoke or drink to excess yourself.

SEE ALSO *Acne vulgaris; Depression; Drugs, misuse of; Parenting; Sex education*

CONTACT **Parentline Plus helpline** 0808 800 2222 (www.parentlineplus.org.uk) **The Brook Advisory Service** 0800 018 5023 (www.brook.org.uk) Confidential contraceptive counselling. **Royal College of Psychiatrists factsheet,** *Surviving adolescence*, is available online at www.rcpsych.ac.uk/info/help/adol/index.asp

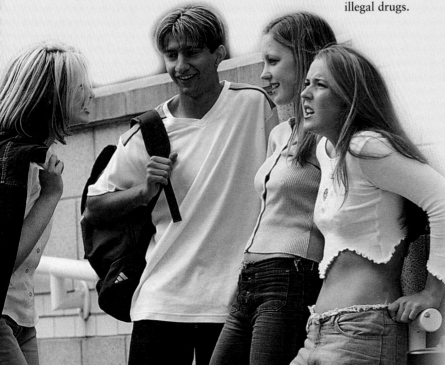

Adrenal glands and disorders

The adrenals are a pair of triangular glands located above the kidneys; they are sometimes referred to as the suprarenal glands. They are responsible for producing hormones that help to regulate the body's chemistry and metabolism and enable us to cope with stress. Each gland has two parts, the outer adrenal cortex surrounding the inner core, the adrenal medulla.

THE ADRENAL CORTEX

More than two dozen steroid hormones (**corticosteroids**) are manufactured by the adrenal cortex. Their production is stimulated by the adrenocorticotropic hormone (ACTH), produced by the pituitary gland. The release of ACTH is in turn triggered by corticotrophin-releasing hormone (CRH), produced by a part of the brain called the hypothalamus.

The cells of the adrenal cortex are arranged in three layers or zones. The *zona glomerulosa*, the outer layer, produces hormones called mineralocorticoids, which control the body's fluid and mineral balance. The main one is aldosterone, which helps the kidneys to retain sodium (salt) and excrete potassium, thereby helping to regulate blood volume and pressure.

The *zona fasciculata*, the middle layer, produces glucocorticoids, the most important of which is cortisol (hydrocortisone). Cortisol has many functions, but one of the most crucial is helping the body to deal with stress and change. Other functions include:
- helping to control fluid levels in the body;
- helping to maintain blood pressure and cardiovascular function;
- modifying the body's response to inflammation;
- stimulating the liver to raise blood glucose levels and balancing the effects of insulin;
- regulating the metabolism of proteins, carbohydrates and fats.

The *zona reticularis*, the cortex's inner layer, also produces glucocorticoids, together with sex hormones (gonadocorticoids). The main ones are androgens (male sex hormones), although small amounts of oestrogens (female sex hormones) are also produced.

THE ADRENAL MEDULLA

The adrenal medulla consists of a mass of neurons (nerve cells) and is strictly speaking part of the body's **autonomic nervous system**, which controls involuntary functions such as breathing and heart rate. The medulla secretes two important hormones, **adrenaline** and noradrenaline, which are involved in activating the body's 'fight or flight' response under stress.

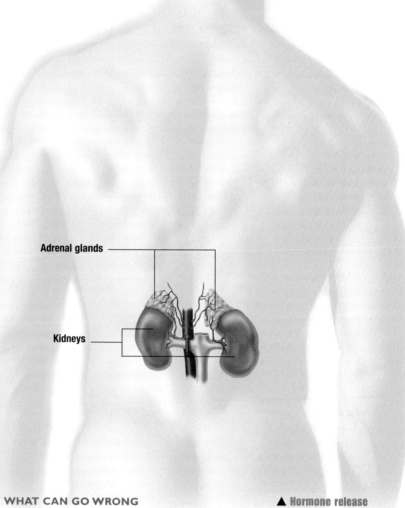

Adrenal glands

Kidneys

WHAT CAN GO WRONG

Problems with the adrenals are rare, but when they occur they may be due to either insufficient production or overproduction of adrenal hormones. Disorders are more likely to affect the cortex than the medulla.

Among the most alarming adrenal disorders is Waterhouse–Frederichsen syndrome. In this disorder, fever, bluish discoloration of the skin (cyanosis) due to insufficient oxygen, and bleeding into the skin from the adrenals are caused by severe meningococcal infection. It is fatal if not treated immediately.

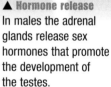

▲ **Hormone release**
In males the adrenal glands release sex hormones that promote the development of the testes.

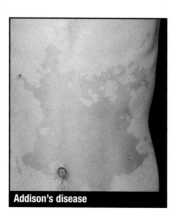

Addison's disease

◄ **Addison's mark**
One symptom of Addison's disease is vitiligo (milk-white patches) in the skin. Other symptoms can include black freckles on the head and neck as well as tiredness and nausea.

Among the disorders that are due to the underproduction of hormones by the adrenal glands is Addison's disease. Problems due to overproduction of hormones include Cushing's syndrome, congenital adrenal hyperplasia and hyperaldosteronism.

Addison's disease

Addison's disease affects three in 100,000 people in the West. In 70 per cent of cases the disease is due to destruction of the adrenal cortex by an **autoimmune disorder** (when the body turns against itself). In the past, tuberculosis (TB) was a major cause, and in the developing world it still is. TB accounts for about one in five cases in the developed world.

Addison's disease may be caused by problems within the adrenal glands themselves, causing underproduction of adrenal hormones. This is known as primary adrenal insufficiency. It may also be caused by a problem such as a tumour affecting the pituitary gland, which causes failure of ACTH production; this is known as secondary adrenal insufficiency.

Symptoms include weight loss, muscle weakness, fatigue, low blood pressure and an increase in skin pigmentation. Symptoms often appear so gradually that they are missed until a stressful event, infection, trauma or operation triggers acute adrenal failure (Addisonian crisis). This causes severe pains in the abdomen and the back of the legs, confusion and loss of consciousness. If left untreated, it can be fatal.

Cushing's syndrome

Cushing's syndrome is a rare condition that results from overproduction of cortisol or other corticoid hormones produced by the adrenal glands. These hormones regulate the use of carbohydrates in the body – an excess upsets the body's regular pattern of converting food into energy.

Symptoms include a rounded 'moon' face, central body fat, muscle wasting, high **blood pressure**, thin skin that bruises easily and reduced resistence to infection. Someone with Cushing's syndrome may also develop glucose intolerance, excessive facial hair, **osteoporosis**, kidney stones, menstrual irregularities or mental health problems such as depression and anxiety.

The disorder may be caused by a problem affecting the adrenals themselves or by excessive secretion of ACTH as a result of a pituitary tumour or, sometimes, by lung or other cancer. It may also be due to overuse of cortisol or other steroid hormones prescribed for the treatment of diseases such as asthma, rheumatoid arthritis, systemic lupus, inflammatory bowel disease and allergies.

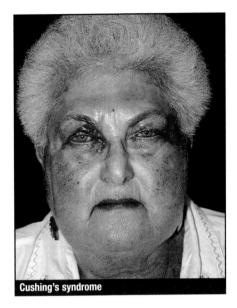

Cushing's syndrome

◀ 'Moon' face
People with Cushing's syndrome, caused by overproduction of corticoid hormones, develop a rounded face as part of general weight gain.

Cushing's disease is a type of Cushing's syndrome due to overproduction of ACTH by the pituitary; indeed, 70 per cent of cases of Cushing's syndrome that occur are caused by pituitary problems.

The underlying causes of Cushing's syndrome are better understood now, which could lead to better diagnosis and treatment. Improved methods of measuring the level of ACTH and other hormones are allowing doctors to distinguish between different causes of Cushing's syndrome.

Some research is looking at the origins of the benign pituitary tumours that underlie most cases of Cushing's. The identification of some faulty genes may provide further clues. Other researchers have discovered that retinoic acid, a derivative of vitamin A, can help to inhibit ACTH production in the laboratory.

Congenital adrenal hyperplasia

Congenital adrenal hyperplasia (CAH), also known as adrenogenital syndrome or adrenal virilism, describes a group of rare inherited disorders that affects around one baby in 10,000 within the UK, both boys and girls. It is caused by the lack of an enzyme needed by the adrenal glands to make the hormones cortisol and aldosterone. It results in the overproduction of androgens (male sex hormones).

In male babies there are no obvious symptoms. However, by the age of two or three, a boy with the condition becomes increasingly muscular, the penis enlarges, pubic hair appears and the voice deepens. In female babies, there is masculinization, including an enlarged clitoris. As the girl grows older she develops a deep voice and facial hair, and fails to ovulate and menstruate.

Some forms of CAH can lead to an adrenal crisis in the newborn baby, causing vomiting, dehydration, changes in fluid and mineral balance and disturbances of heart rhythm.

Developments in hormonal and DNA testing could revolutionize detection and diagnosis of congenital adrenal hyperplasia. For example, a heel-prick test can now be carried out on babies in the first week of life that is designed to detect hormonal markers in the blood. This replaces older, slower methods of testing and enables newborn boys who have CAH but exhibit no symptoms to be diagnosed early, thereby avoiding a life-threatening adrenal crisis. Meanwhile, ever more sophisticated gene technology is paving the way for prenatal and neonatal screening.

Hyperaldosteronism

Hyperaldosteronism is caused by excessive production of the hormone aldosterone, which controls the body's water balance. The most commonly known form of the disorder is Conn's syndrome in which, in many cases, the only symptom is raised **blood pressure**, but there may also be excessive thirst and an increased production of urine.

The condition is diagnosed by blood and urine tests. Its underlying cause – which may or may not be a problem affecting the adrenals themselves – needs to be identified and treated.

Tumours affecting the adrenal glands

Occasionally, a benign (non-cancerous) or malignant (cancerous) tumour may develop in the adrenal glands. Some tumours affect production of hormones – causing either underproduction or, more commonly, overproduction – but in many cases hormone production is unaffected.

Tumours that do not affect hormone production are found only by accident when the person is tested for another illness or condition.

PHAEOCHROMOCYTOMA

A phaeochromocytoma is a rare cancer that often begins inside a group of cells known as chromaffin cells in the adrenal medulla. One of its effects is to cause overproduction of adrenaline and noradrenaline, leading to symptoms of high **blood pressure**, headaches, sweating, pounding of the heart, pain in the chest and a feeling of anxiety.

Phaeochromocytoma is sometimes part of a syndrome called multiple endocrine neoplasia (MEN) in which there is thyroid cancer and other hormonal problems.

CANCER OF THE ADRENAL CORTEX

Cancer of the adrenal cortex is a rare form of cancer that can cause either overproduction

or underproduction of hormones, leading to a wide range of symptoms including high blood pressure, osteoporosis, diabetes or changes in sexual characteristics such as deepening of the voice, excessive hairiness (hirsutism), swelling of the clitoris or of the breasts. Other symptoms include pain in the abdomen, loss of weight without dieting, and weakness.

NEUROBLASTOMA

A neuroblastoma is a solid tumour affecting nerve tissue that generally begins in the adrenal glands. Children under the age of five are most commonly affected. Symptoms include protruding eyes and dark circles around the eyes.

CONTACT **Addison's Disease Self-help Group** Contact Deana Kenward (01483) 830673 (www.adshg.org.uk)
Association for Cushing's Treatment and Help Contact Elaine Eldridge (01628) 670389
The Pituitary Foundation PO Box 1944, Bristol BS99 2UB 0845 450 0375 (www.pituitary.org.uk)
Climb Climb Building, 176 Nantwich Road, Crewe CW2 6BG (01270) 257141 (www.climb.org.uk) Deals with more than 730 inherited metabolic diseases affecting children

Adrenaline

Adrenaline is one of the two main 'stress' hormones produced by the **adrenal glands**; the other is noradrenaline. Adrenaline increases the heart rate and the force with which the heart pumps. It increases the flow of blood to the muscles and brain, constricts blood vessels in the skin and gut (allowing more blood to be available for use by the muscles), relaxes the smooth muscles and helps to convert the stored **carbohydrate** glycogen to glucose for instant energy.

Synthetic adrenaline may be injected to treat **anaphylactic shock**, an acute **asthma** attack or a **cardiac arrest**. Adrenaline eyedrops are used to treat **glaucoma**.
SEE ALSO **Stress**

Adrenocorticotropic hormone

Adrenocorticotropic hormone (ACTH), also called corticotrophin, is a hormone that stimulates the **adrenal glands** to produce corticosteroid hormones, which help the body to deal with stress. ACTH is produced by the pituitary gland disorders, and production is triggered by the release of corticotrophin-releasing hormone (CRH), produced by the hypothalamus, a region of the brain that coordinates the nervous and hormonal systems.

Levels of ACTH fluctuate with the body's daily rhythm, peaking in the morning after getting up.

Advance directive

An advance directive, also known as a living will, is a signed statement of healthcare preferences. It can be referred to if someone is no longer able to express his or her wishes due to physical or mental illness, injury, dementia or confusion. Usually it makes statements about accepting or refusing medical treatment, although such requests may not be carried out despite the person's intentions and preparations.
SEE ALSO *Death and dying*

Aerobic exercise

Aerobic exercise is any sustained activity that forces the body to increase its consumption of oxygen. Brisk walking, running, cycling, swimming, rowing and dancing are all forms of aerobic exercise. Such exercise improves cardiovascular fitness by strengthening the heart, improving oxygen circulation and boosting respiration. Aerobic exercise develops stamina (the ability to keep going) by training the heart, lungs and circulation system to improve the delivery of oxygen to the muscles.
SEE ALSO *Anaerobic exercise; Exercise and health*

Affective disorder

The word affective means relating to mood, so the term affective disorder covers a range of problems including mania, mood swings, depression and manic depression. There is also a condition known as schizoaffective disorder in which some symptoms of schizophrenia and those of a mood disorder are combined.

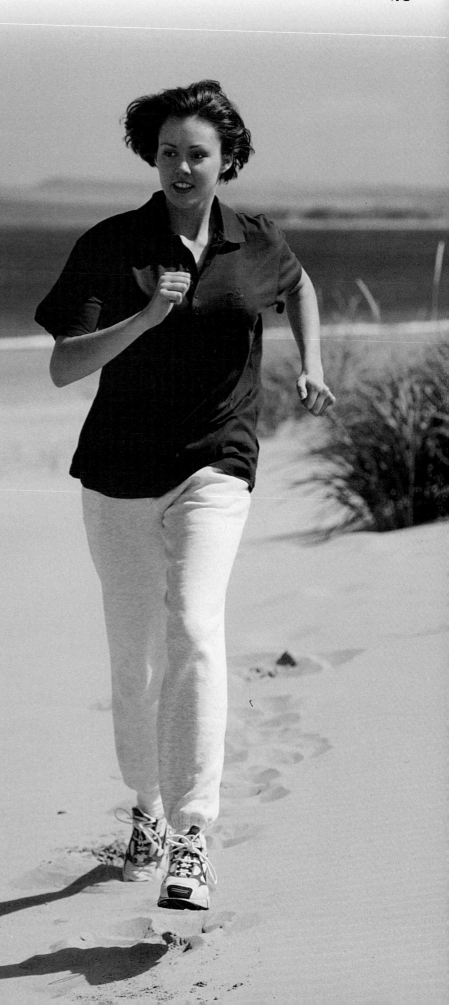

▶ **Aerobic exercise**
Moderate aerobic exercise is important in order to maintain good health and build up physical stamina.

Age and ageing

Average life expectancy, medicine and health care have improved dramatically since the beginning of the 20th century, bringing many advantages, but there are also some disadvantages.

Improved health and increased life expectancy have created many opportunities for people to add a new dimension to their later years. Life beyond the age of 60 need no longer be regarded as slowing down and growing old but it has to be recognized that living longer does not guarantee living in good health. However, advances in medicine mean that we are better equipped than we used to be to cope with many of the conditions that affect older people. Following a healthy lifestyle and being aware of the various ailments and symptoms that could strike us at different stages in our lives improves our resistance to disease and increases the chances of spotting problems before they develop into potentially life-threatening conditions.

Babies, for example, are particularly prone to many illnesses as their immune system develops, including colds, eczema and colic (see **Babies and baby care**). Children are more likely to suffer infectious diseases such as chickenpox. This may be because schoolchildren are more frequently exposed to potential infection and their bodies have not yet built up resistance to these germs. Teenagers are more vulnerable than adults to conditions such as glandular fever or tonsillitis.

As people progress into middle age and later life, they are more likely to encounter problems such as **osteoporosis** (a thinning of the bones that may lead to fractures), various **cancers** and osteoarthritis (inflammation of the joints caused by 'wear and tear', as the protective cartilage space between the bones of the joints wears away with age – see **Arthritis**).

Growing old is characterized by a natural, progressive decline in the body's systems. Every part of the body is affected: among other changes, hair turns grey, skin wrinkles, joints and muscles lose flexibility, bones become weak, memory declines, eyesight diminishes, and immunity is impaired.

There are several theories about what makes human beings age, but none of them has been proven. One theory is that ageing is predetermined by genes that affect the rate at which cells die; as cells die off, organs begin to malfunction and eventually cannot maintain the biological functions necessary to sustain life. Another theory argues that chemical reactions between cells in the body cause toxins called 'free radicals' to form; the free radicals then damage the cells, causing a person to age.

▼ **In the swim**
As we grow older, our metabolism slows down and our energy needs decrease – so regular exercise is vital to avoid excess weight and maintain fitness.

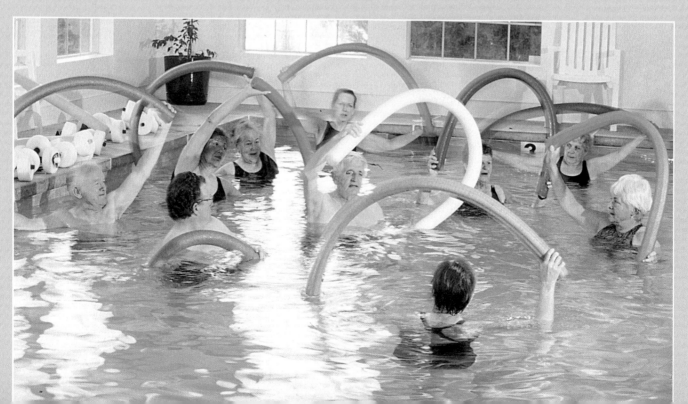

THE AGEING PROCESS

One of the first common signs of ageing occurs when people reach their early 40s. The lens in each eye becomes increasingly stiff, and focusing on close objects becomes difficult, a problem known as long-sightedness, or presbyopia. A deterioration in hearing (presbyacusis) may also occur, due to the loss of hair cells in the cochlea, the part of the ear that processes sounds for the brain to interpret. This reduces the ability to hear the highest-pitched tones – so that even clearly pronounced speech is perceived as mumbling.

Most internal organs are affected by ageing. The more often cells divide – which they do during growth or when damaged – the more vulnerable they are to developing abnormally or not at all. Some cells are programmed to reproduce a fixed number of times and then die, by a process known as apoptosis. Research has shown that these cells can not reproduce indefinitely because the endcaps on each DNA strand, known as telomeres, shorten with each cell divide. At some point, the telomere is reduced to nothing and the cell can no longer divide. It then becomes a junk cell which interferes with other cells causing them to deteriorate. Cells such as nerve, kidney and heart muscle cells do not reproduce – so when they are lost through wear and tear, they are not replaced. Sometimes cells undergo DNA changes, known as mutations, that make them behave abnormally, and a cancer may develop.

It is usually disease, rather than the ageing process itself, that is more damaging to health. The gradual decline in internal bodily functions means that older people are more susceptible both to illness and to adverse effects of drugs.

Distribution of body fat also changes in later life – there is less fat under the skin and more in the abdominal area, so the skin becomes thinner and more fragile and body shape changes.

AVOIDING DISEASE IN LATER LIFE

Certain health problems are more likely to occur in later life, and some conditions are confined almost exclusively to older adults. Apart from osteoporosis and osteoarthritis, these include **cataracts, glaucoma, prostate cancer, Alzheimer's disease** and other **dementias**, urinary **incontinence** and **strokes**.

However, there is a lot we can do to prevent the onset of disease and maximize our quality of life. For people who smoke, the single biggest step to improving health, whatever your age, is to stop **smoking**. This not only reduces your chances of developing coronary heart disease, lung cancer and other respiratory problems, but also slows down the rate at which the skin ages. Regular exercise, good nutrition and sufficient sleep are other important factors in disease prevention.

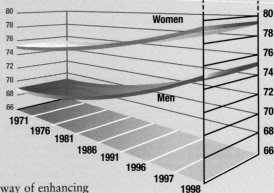

▶ **Living longer**
Life expectancy in the UK has risen steadily since the 1970s for women (shown in pink) and men (blue). Women can still generally expect to live longer than men.

KEEPING ACTIVE

Exercise is an effective way of enhancing health. It not only helps to strengthen the lungs and cardiovascular system but also reduces the risk of osteoporosis by strengthening the bones, keeps the body supple and helps to maintain a healthy body weight. This in turn reduces the risk of heart disease. Taking exercise can also be fun.

Age is usually no barrier to taking up a physical activity, but anyone embarking on a new exercise programme should consult a doctor first. If you are 75 years old or over, you are entitled to an annual NHS health check, especially if you are having medical treatment or experiencing mobility problems, in which case your doctor or physiotherapist can help you with an exercise programme or suggest a class. Some GPs offer 'prescriptions for health' – often referred to as 'GP referral schemes' – in which they may prescribe, for example, a course of supervised exercise for a condition to be undertaken at a sports centre.

There are many other ways to keep fit. People who like solitary activity could take up walking, cycling or swimming. If you like company, a wide range of classes and clubs is on offer, which also provide a way of meeting like-minded people. Many local authorities run classes for older people, and some are specifically for those with medical conditions such as heart disease and arthritis. An organization called EXTEND provides 'movement to music' classes for anyone aged 60 or over. Local libraries, sports centres or council offices can provide information for your area. (See also **Exercise and health**.)

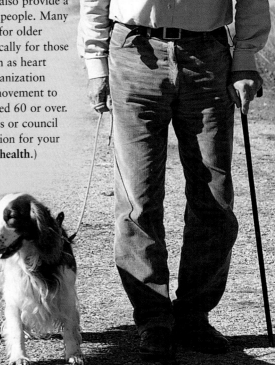

▶ **Enjoyable activity**
To promote good health, doctors recommend that all adults take moderate exercise for no less than 30 minutes a day on at least five days a week.

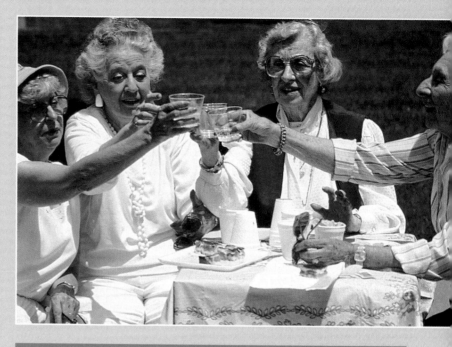

▶ **Liquid intake**
The amount of fluid needed by the body remains the same throughout adult life. Whatever your age, you should aim to drink six to eight glasses of water a day.

MAINTAINING A HEALTHY DIET

Most of us find that our energy requirements decrease with age, but continuing to keep active will help you to maintain a good appetite – which in turn helps to ensure an adequate intake of essential vitamins and minerals (see **Diet**). Older people must take care to drink enough fluids to avoid **dehydration**, which may in turn cause mental confusion.

Some nutrients are particularly important in later life. These include calcium, which may help to reduce bone loss, and vitamin D, which is necessary for calcium absorption. Exposure to sunlight helps the body to produce vitamin D so housebound people are particularly at risk of deficiency. Nutritionists recommend that everyone over the age of 65 years takes a supplement of vitamin D and includes food sources such as oily fish and margarine in their diet. (See **Nutritional supplements**.)

HORMONE REPLACEMENT THERAPY

HRT can relieve menopausal symptoms and problems such as hot flushes and osteoporosis. Long-term usage has been described as giving a feeling of youthful well-being. However, if taken long term HRT gives a small increased risk of certain cancers, particularly breast cancer, and there seem to be no benefits for heart disease as was hoped. Many doctors advise HRT only for short periods, as the long-term risks can outweigh the benefits. If you are thinking of taking HRT, it is important to talk with your doctor.

SLEEPING WELL

A good night's sleep plays a vital part in the body's repair process. Lack of sleep can be a factor in a variety of ailments, ranging from loss of energy to depression (see **Sleep and disorders**). Chronic sleep deprivation can compromise the immune system and make a person more susceptible to infections.

The amount of sleep each person needs varies widely, ranging from three to eleven hours per night. Most people need less sleep as they get older but they should have enough sleep to feel refreshed. If you avoid naps during the day, it is more likely that you will achieve a satisfactory amount of sleep at night. Keeping active also tends to promote a good quality and quantity of sleep, as does sleeping in a warm, comfortable bed.

Preventing health problems with supplements

A range of daily vitamin and mineral supplements will improve general health and can help to prevent specific disorders.

AILMENT	PREVENTION
Recurrent upper respiratory tract infections	Daily multivitamin and multimineral complex; daily amount as directed on the label.
Congestive heart failure	Vitamin B complex (50–1000mcg vitamin B_{12}, 400mcg folic acid and 50mg vitamin B_6 daily).
Osteoporosis	Daily supplements of marine fish oils, evening primrose oil with calcium, or calcium (1g daily) and vitamin D (400 IU/10mcg daily).
Heart rhythm disturbance	Magnesium supplement (300mg daily) and daily multivitamins.
Muscle cramps	Magnesium supplement (300mg daily), calcium supplement (500mg twice a day) and daily multivitamins.
High blood pressure	Vitamin C supplement (1g daily) to help to reduce stroke risk, and magnesium supplement (300mg) to help to lower blood pressure, especially in women.
Cardiovascular disease	Vitamin E supplement (600 IU/400mg daily), but not if taking the anticoagulant warfarin, and vitamic C (1g daily).
Complications of diabetes	Chromium supplement (200mcg daily) if mildly diabetic, subject to approval by a doctor.
Memory loss	120mg ginkgo biloba daily, if not on anticoagulants.

SUPPORT AND BENEFITS

Anyone aged 60 or over is entitled to receive free medicines in the UK and, at 65 or over, you are entitled to free flu vaccinations. Free annual health checks are available to people over 75 years. These checks may include an assessment of the person's mental and physical health, including mobility, continence, hearing and eyesight, and a review of diet, use of medicines, accommodation, family support and social links.

Older people who come to find it difficult to cope with living at home can arrange for additional services or care to make life easier. Depending on where you live, health authorities, housing departments, social services departments and charities provide a range of services.

Alternatively, you may decide that moving into sheltered housing or into a nursing or residential home is the best option.

SEE ALSO *Accident prevention; Blood pressure and problems; Community care; Ear and problems; Eye and problems; Diet; Heart and circulatory system; Home care and nursing; Memory loss and distortion; Muscular system; Respiratory system*

CONTACT **Age Concern** For England Astral House, 1268 London Road, London SW16 4ER (020) 8765 7200 (www.ageconcern.org.uk); **For Wales** 4th Floor, 1 Cathedral Road, Cardiff CF11 9SD (029) 2037 1566 (www.accymru. org. uk); **For Scotland,** 113 Rose Street, Edinburgh EH2 3DT (0131) 220 3345 (www.ageconcernscotland. org.uk) **For N. Ireland** 3 Lower Crescent, Belfast BT7 1NR (028) 9024 5729 Offers help on lifestyles, communities, social interaction and many other issues.
Counsel and Care Twyman House, 16 Bonny Street, London NW1 9PG 0845 300 7585 10am–1pm (Mon–Fri) (www.counselandcare. org.uk) Information for the over 60s, their carers, friends, relatives and professionals.
EXTEND 2 Place Farm, Wheathampstead, Herts AL4 8SB (01582) 832760 (www.extend.org.uk) Movement to music classes for over 60s and the less able of any age.
Help the Aged For England 207–221 Pentonville Road, London N1 9UZ (020) 7278 1114; **For Scotland** 11 Granton Square, Edinburgh (0131) 551 6331; **For Wales** 12 Cathedral Road, Cardiff, CF11 9LJ (02920) 390 898; **For N. Ireland** Ascot House, Shaftesbury Square, Belfast BT2 7DB (02890) 248 183 (www.helptheaged.org.uk) Produces a wide range of material for older people from money matters to housing to health.

Agoraphobia

Agoraphobia is the term used for a group of **phobias** (intense fears) that includes fear of open spaces, crowded places, being alone, or being in any place where sufferers believe that they are likely to experience panic.

Agoraphobia is common – an estimated 13 per cent of the UK population suffer from some form of it. More women seek help for it than men. The condition, which usually starts during the late teenage years or in the early 20s, may either arise after a frightening event or seem to come from nowhere. You may be more vulnerable to developing agoraphobia if someone in your family has the condition.

SYMPTOMS

The characteristics of agoraphobia include feelings of anxiety and panic such as rapid heartbeat, churning stomach, sweating or a dry mouth, which occur when the sufferer is alone, away from home, in crowds or in public places.

People with agoraphobia attempt to avoid situations associated with earlier panic attacks because of their intense fear that the attacks will recur.

TREATMENT

Someone who is afflicted by agoraphobia should seek help as early as possible. Join a self-help group for support and to learn coping strategies. Consult a doctor if symptoms worsen or the condition becomes unmanageable.

What a doctor may do

People suffering from agoraphobia may be referred to a psychologist for **behaviour therapy** or **cognitive behaviour therapy**. They may be prescribed **antidepressants** or **tranquillizers** for a short time.

Complementary therapies

The following may help to ease symptoms:
- therapies such as **massage** or **aromatherapy** to help you to relax;
- **hypnotherapy.**

SEE ALSO *Anxiety; Obsessions and compulsions; Panic attack; Phobia*

CONTACT **National Phobics Society** Zion Community Resource Centre, 339 Stretford Road, Hulme, Manchester M15 4ZY; helpline 0870 770 0456 (www.phobics-society.org.uk) **Triumph over Phobia (TOP UK)** PO Box 344, Bristol BS34 8ZR 0845 600 9601 (www.triumphoverphobia.com) **Mind** 15–19 Broadway, London E15 4BQ; Mind*info*line 0845 766 0163 9.15am–5.15pm Mon–Fri (www.mind.org.uk) Campaigns for better mental health services.

AIDS

AIDS stands for Acquired Immune Deficiency Syndrome, a disease caused by infection with **HIV** (human immunodeficiency virus). The HIV virus can be caught through contact with certain bodily fluids of an infected person.

Saliva, sweat and urine do not usually contain enough HIV to infect another person. The most common method by which the virus is passed is during sexual intercourse, both heterosexual and homosexual; from mother to baby before or during birth or during breastfeeding; and when injecting drug abusers share needles and other equipment. It is also possible for HIV to be transmitted through organ **transplants, blood transfusion** and the use of blood products; this is rare in the UK because donated blood and tissue are screened for the virus.

SYMPTOMS

When first infected with HIV, some people may notice a brief flu-like illness, but most people are not aware that they have become infected and will have no symptoms for many years. However, once they are infectious, their immune system starts to make antibodies to the virus straight away. When these antibodies are detected by blood testing, people are said to be HIV-positive. Gradually the virus attacks the body's immune system, making it hard for the person to resist infection.

The CD4 T-lymphocyte cells in the blood are particularly prone to attack by the HIV virus (see **Immune system and disorders**). These are helper cells that organize the body's response to viral invasion. A normal T-lymphocyte count is 500–1500/ml blood (1fl oz = 28ml). AIDS has developed once the T-lymphocyte count has dropped below 200ml and the person is suffering weight loss, diarrhoea, fever, certain types of pneumonia and skin cancer. Damage to the immune system, skin or other defences makes the person also subject to infection with Candida (see **Fungal infections**) or **cytomegalovirus**. People with this test result and the described symptoms are said to have full-blown AIDS.

TREATMENT

If you suspect that you may be infected with the HIV virus, contact your local genito-urinary medicine (GUM) clinic to arrange a test. These are run by your health authority and are usually attached to a general hospital. Many treatments now available can decrease the rate of progress of HIV and alleviate many of the symptoms, but there is as yet no cure for AIDS.

CONTACT **Terrence Higgins Trust** 0845 122 1200 (www.tht.org.uk)

Albinism

Albinism is a condition that prevents the production of the brown pigment melanin, normally found in the skin, hair and eyes. As a result, people with albinism have very pale skin and hair. Their eyes appear pink because of the colour of the blood vessels at the back of the eye, which are normally masked by melanin.

Albinism is fairly common, affecting about one in every 20,000 children born worldwide. It can be a serious health problem in hot countries, where many albinos die of skin cancer in their teens or twenties. They also frequently suffer social ostracism as a consequence of their pale skins. Albinism also occurs in animals.

SYMPTOMS

■ Pale skin, white hair and pink eyes.
■ Defective eyesight in people with oculo-cutaneous albinism, the commonest form of albinism. This is because the absence of melanin prevents the optic nerve from developing properly when babies are in the womb.
■ Susceptibility to sunburn, due to lack of the normal protection provided by melanin.

CAUSES

Albinism is the result of several different genetic mutations, which may be inherited or may occur spontaneously. The condition prevents or restricts the ability to produce melanin.

COMPLICATIONS

People with albinism have a higher than average risk of developing skin cancers.

SEE ALSO *Genetics and genetic disorders*

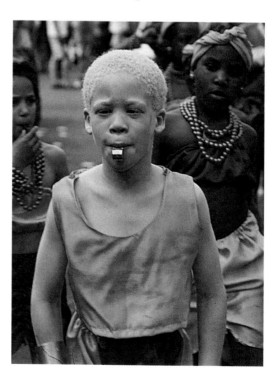

◀ **Skin deep**
In Africa and other parts of the world where most native people have dark skin and hair, albinos can be affected by social discrimination and prejudice.

Alcohol and abuse

Moderate consumption of alcohol promotes relaxation and offers a range of health benefits. But alcohol abuse – when intake rises above moderate levels – presents a severe health risk and can cause great misery.

Pure alcohol is a colourless, volatile and flammable liquid produced by the fermentation of sugars and starches. It can be used as a solvent or antiseptic as well as a recreational drug in alcoholic drinks. Historically, people have found alcoholic drinks useful for their pain-relieving, tonic and medicinal properties, and for promoting social interaction, sleep and relaxation. Alcohol played a vital health role in the early development of towns and cities, when mild alcoholic beverages were much safer to drink than sewage-polluted water.

HARMFUL EFFECTS OF ALCOHOL

There are many dangers associated with excessive consumption of alcohol. Some are directly linked to drinking, others are subtle consequences of the damage alcohol can cause. Health risks include the following.

- Red wine may cause migraine in some susceptible individuals.
- Alcohol causes weight gain and obesity – it is high in calories with little nutritional value.
- Nutritional imbalances are caused if drinking interferes with a proper diet.
- Alcohol can interfere with normal liver function. Cirrhosis of the liver affects one in five heavy drinkers.
- Alcohol may cause **blood pressure** to rise, which is linked to the risk of coronary artery disease and **stroke**.
- Alcohol may be dangerous if it is mixed with some medications.
- Alcohol can provoke melancholy or aggression.
- Frequent drinkers risk developing problem drinking and alcohol dependence (see page 88).
- Pregnant women who drink heavily may cause their baby to be born with **fetal alcohol syndrome**. Consumption of more than 56 units a week in pregnancy can lead to low birth weight, cleft palate and mental retardation.
- Heavy consumption of alcohol is linked with **infertility**.
- Excessive drinking leads to increased risk of **cancers** of the mouth, throat, gullet, stomach and liver, and possibly also breast and colon.

In the UK, 65–80 per cent of assault victims needing hospital treatment are intoxicated at the time of injury.

Checklist

Follow common-sense guidelines to avoid problems associated with alcohol.

Do

- ✔ Enjoy socializing with friends.
- ✔ Watch your limits (see Sensible drinking, page 86).
- ✔ Drink plenty of water as well as alcohol.
- ✔ Try to encourage sensible attitudes to drinking in children.

Don't

- ✘ Drink and drive.
- ✘ Operate dangerous machinery after drinking.
- ✘ Drink on an empty stomach.
- ✘ Drink before swimming or playing physical sports where there is a risk of injury.
- ✘ Drink before climbing ladders or undertaking other hazardous activities.
- ✘ Drink while taking incompatible medication.
- ✘ Binge drink (consume large amounts of alcohol occasionally).

Heavy alcohol consumption is connected to social problems such as vandalism, delinquency, petty crime, absenteeism and reduced performance at work, and unnecessary use of NHS resources.

In the UK alcohol use is associated with:
- 20–30 per cent of accidents;
- 40 per cent of crimes such as assault and mugging;
- 50 per cent of assaults in the home;
- 65 per cent of suicide attempts;
- 60–70 per cent of murders;
- 70 per cent of beatings;
- 75 per cent of stabbings.

MODERATE CONSUMPTION

Doctors now recognize that there are broad health benefits from moderate alcohol consumption – up to four units daily.

Research shows that drinking moderate amounts of alcohol reduces the risk of coronary artery disease and offers protection against arteriosclerosis. Moderate drinking also reduces the likelihood of blood clots in the blood vessels or heart.

Alcoholic drinks contain **antioxidants**, which may protect against some cancers. Red wine may help to reduce the risk of **Alzheimer's disease**.

> Some 94 per cent of young people in the UK have tried alcohol by age 16. The peak age for arrests for drunkenness is 18.

Drinking moderate amounts of alcohol also has certain nutritional benefits. It increases levels of 'good' lipids in the blood (see **Cholesterol**). Red wine and beer contain the B vitamin complex and some minerals.

ALCOHOL AND YOUNG PEOPLE

Young people drink less often than adults, but tend to binge drink (see below). This can lead to health problems due to intoxication, accidents, unsafe sex and crime.

Children and most adolescents have smaller body structures than adults and are likely to get drunk more quickly. They are less able to absorb the alcohol: if they drink heavily they are more likely to suffer from alcoholic poisoning, and have a higher risk of slipping into a coma and experiencing metabolic disturbances and breathing difficulties as a result.

Research shows that young people in Britain are starting to drink unsupervised at an earlier age and are drinking a greater quantity than ever before. Moreover, they are now more likely to be drinking spirit-based drinks. Reasons for these developments include peer pressure; curiosity about alcohol and its effects; wanting to appear grown-up; lack of experience with alcohol; lack of role models for sensible drinking; media images of alcohol as glamorous; and the promotion of alcoholic drinks specifically targeted at the young.

What parents can do

The age at which children first experience alcohol is less important than when they begin unsupervised drinking. In France, children often drink watered-down wine with family meals from an early age. Introducing children to alcohol within the home serves to fulfil their curiosity in a safe setting and to encourage sensible attitudes towards drinking.

Parents can also help children to develop a responsible attitude to alcohol by being good role models for sensible drinking. The children of heavy drinkers – and of teetotallers – are more likely to develop alcohol problems than the children of moderate drinkers.

Adults in a position to influence children should not drink to excess, and should never drink and drive. They should be willing to discuss attitudes to alcohol with children, and should ensure that a child's first experiences with alcohol are supervised. If you do allow children to drink alcohol, do so only with meals, and water the drink down.

Binge drinking

Many people – especially young men, but increasingly young women also – concentrate their drinking into sessions once or twice a week. Such 'binge drinking' is more dangerous to health than drinking the same number of units more evenly spaced throughout the week. Binge

Factfile

Sensible drinking

Moderate alcohol consumption does have some health benefits. People who drink moderately live longer than teetotallers but regularly drinking more than the recommended amount has greater health disadvantages. 1 unit of alcohol is equivalent to a small glass of wine, half a pint of beer, a small glass of sherry or port or a standard pub measure of spirits, but remember that a drink poured at home is likely to be bigger than a pub measure.

Safe daily intake: Women 2–3 units   Men 3–4 units

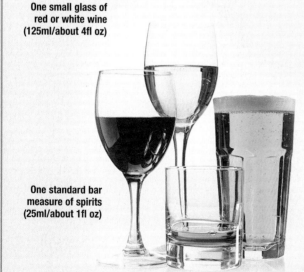

One small glass of red or white wine (125ml/about 4fl oz)

Half a pint of average-strength beer (250ml)

One standard bar measure of spirits (25ml/about 1fl oz)

How alcohol affects the body

Alcohol is absorbed into the bloodstream between 15 and 90 minutes after drinking, depending on the contents of the stomach. On average, it takes one hour per unit for alcohol to be broken down in the liver. The immediate physical effects of alcohol are listed below.

- Depressed activity of the central nervous system.
- Faster heart rate.
- Slower reaction time.
- Impaired judgment.
- Reduced coordination.
- Loss of inhibitions.

As a person gets drunker, effects include:

- Dehydration.
- Slurred speech.
- Clumsiness.
- Loss of balance.
- Blurring of vision.
- Unconsciousness.

The effects of alcohol are greater:

- For people of small build and low weight.
- For women – because they metabolize alcohol more slowly than men.
- For the very young or very old.
- For some Orientals who metabolize alcohol less readily than Caucasians.
- When drinking on an empty stomach.

You may still be over the limit for safe driving the morning after late-night heavy drinking.

drinking may precipitate **gout**, lead to a heart attack, provoke pancreatitis, increase risks of liver damage, and disturb heart rhythm. Binge drinking can also, very rarely, prove fatal (for example, by causing heart failure or by suffocation when people choke on their own vomit). Binge drinking leads to a level of drunkenness that can cause a serious accident.

PROBLEM DRINKING AND CHILDREN

Children of problem drinkers often have difficulty with their self-esteem and are less likely to achieve their potential both in their childhood and later in life. They are more likely than other children to underachieve at school, to have emotional and psychological problems, and to have difficulties making friends. They are also more likely to exhibit antisocial behaviour and to suffer from a psychiatric disorder. As they grow older they have a higher than normal risk of developing alcohol problems of their own, of involvement with illicit drug-taking and of becoming dependent on either alcohol or drugs.

SOCIAL DRINKING OR PROBLEM DRINKING?

There are several warning signs that drinking is getting out of control. You should consider cutting down if you find that you are using alcohol to deal with stress and crises, are organizing your life around the availability of alcohol, or are having frequent hangovers. Friends, relatives or colleagues might notice obsessive attitudes towards alcohol in a frequent heavy drinker.

Common signs of problem drinking are regular absences from work because of hangovers, family conflicts after drinking, and financial difficulties caused by spending money on drink. Other signs that drinking has become a problem include accidents or injuries due to drinking, forgetting what happened during drinking sessions, and feelings of anger, denial or guilt when others comment on alcohol intake or behaviour.

As well as the potential for causing health problems, financial difficulties, job loss, family breakdown and criminal involvement, there is the possibility that – for about one in 20 of those affected – problem drinking will lead to alcohol dependence (see page 88).

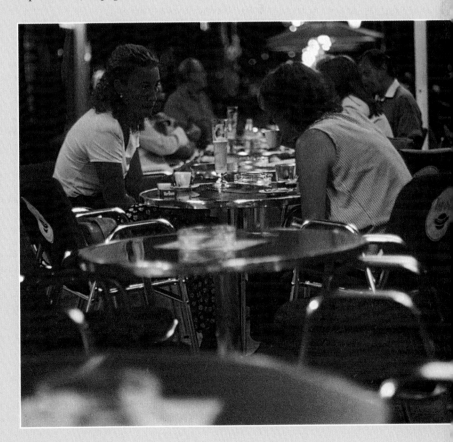

▼ **Over the limit**
For many people alcohol is an essential ingredient in their social life and entertainment. But 33 per cent of men and 20 per cent of women in the UK drink more than the recommended amount of alcohol.

Alcohol dependence

A drinking habit that has developed into an addiction is known as alcohol dependence.

An alcoholic, or alcohol-dependent person, is physically dependent on alcohol. If intake is not maintained, unpleasant withdrawal symptoms result and the person must drink compulsively to avoid them. Withdrawal symptoms include bodily tremors ('the shakes'), anxiety and restlessness, sweating, delusions, hallucinations and delirium.

People with drinking problems that have reached this stage are unlikely to be able to stop drinking unaided, and will need professional help to conquer their addiction. They will usually have to abstain totally from alcohol for the rest of their lives – there is a high risk of relapse into alcoholism with even 'one little drink'.

RECOGNIZING ALCOHOL DEPENDENCE
Signs of possible addiction to alcohol include waking up feeling shaky and sweaty; needing a drink in the morning; needing to drink more to achieve the same effect; and drinking large quantities without feeling drunk. Many of the indicators of problem drinking (see page 87) may also be signs of developing alcohol dependence.
Alcohol dependence in someone else
Most problem drinkers deny their problem. If you are concerned about someone else's drinking, signs to watch for include changes in mood and behaviour, memory lapses or confusion about recent conversations and events, unreliability at work or at home, drinking alone or in secret and lying about drinking, neglecting their personal appearance, trembling hands and regular vomiting.

SEEKING PROFESSIONAL HELP
Help with alcohol dependence is available in the UK through the NHS, voluntary organizations and private clinics. Most of these organizations will offer support and advice to the family and friends of alcoholics as well as to the problem drinkers themselves. Treatment aims include minimizing the damage that the alcoholic is inflicting on others. If you think you, a friend or a relative may be an alcoholic, consider contacting advice lines and counselling services. You could call your GP, who may refer you to an NHS centre. There are also a number of private detoxification and rehabilitation clinics.

TREATMENT OF ALCOHOL DEPENDENCE
The first priority is to get the alcoholic through the symptoms of physical withdrawal when intake is stopped (see **Detoxification**). This process often involves residential treatment.

The next phase is to devise a strategy to help the problem drinker to avoid relapse. Ways of helping a recovering alcoholic to stay off alcohol include **counselling, cognitive behaviour therapy,** self-help groups such as Alcoholics Anonymous (see box) and aversion therapy.

HOW TO HELP AN ALCOHOLIC
The only person who has control over a problem drinker's drinking is the problem drinker, but you can encourage and support his or her efforts to get better. Discuss the problem when the drinker is sober. Try to discover the reasons for drinking and focus on the effects of drinking on his or her life. Encourage the drinker to take responsibility for his or her behaviour and to seek help from a professional or a support group.

Never bail a problem drinker out of problems caused by drink – don't lend money or make excuses for him or her. If the problem drinker is your spouse or a close relative, be sure to take care of yourself, maintain separate interests and seek support outside the relationship.

SEE ALSO *Addictions; Arteries and disorders; Blood and disorders; Diet; Drugs, misuse of; Heart and circulatory system; Liver and disorders; Pancreas and disorders*

CONTACT **Drinkline** – free government helpline for advice on problem drinking 0800 917 8282
Alcohol Concern – web site includes online directory of alcohol treatment services in the UK (www.alcoholconcern.org.uk)
Advice and Counselling on Alcohol and Drugs (ACAD) – charity offering free advice, information and counselling (www.acad.org.uk)
Alcoholics Anonymous 0845 769 7555. There is an unofficial web site with a search facility for local groups (www.alcoholics-anonymous.org.uk)
Al-Anon Family Group UK & Eire 61 Great Dover Street, London SE1 4YF (020) 7403 0888 (www.al-anonuk.org.uk)
The Portman Group – drinks industry-sponsored group to promote enjoyment of alcohol within sensible drinking guidelines (www.portman-group.org.uk)

Factfile
Alcoholics Anonymous (AA)

AA is a worldwide network that offers support for maintaining recovery from alcohol dependence.

Its philosophy requires total abstinence from alcohol and the acceptance of the '12 Steps' – a series of slogans and affirmations. These require AA members to acknowledge a 'higher power', admit their problem and discuss it openly at group meetings.

The 12-Step process is not suitable for everyone, but it can be a powerful aid to maintaining abstinence and has been successfully copied by other groups such as Gamblers Anonymous. Support for families is provided through a network called Al-Anon.

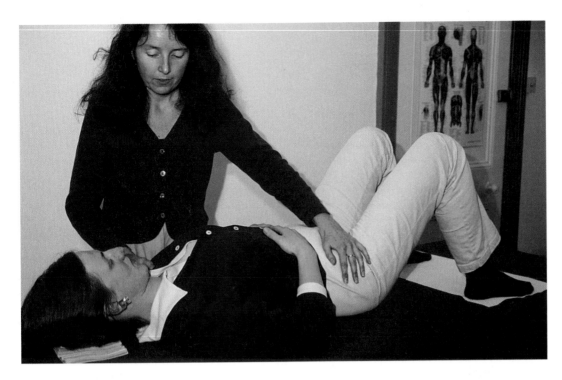

◀ **Correcting posture**
One of the lessons of the Alexander technique focuses on how to lie down with the head supported at a height that follows the natural curve of the spine. This practice encourages the release of tension in the spine and promotes regular breathing.

Alexander technique

The Alexander technique is a gentle system of exercises designed to help people to develop good postural habits. Proponents claim that it alleviates some posture-related health problems.

The Alexander technique is based on the idea that there are correct and incorrect ways of moving, sitting and standing. It was developed in the late 19th century by an Australian actor called Frederick Matthias Alexander after he discovered that changing his posture affected his voice. His techniques, which broadly involve keeping the neck and spine in line, aim to eradicate 'old patterns of misuse' in the body.

WHAT IT IS USED FOR
- Breathing problems.
- Back, neck and joint pain.
- Fatigue, anxiety, stress and headaches.
- To promote self-awareness and confidence.

ORTHODOX VIEW
The Alexander technique is accepted by most doctors. It is available on the NHS in some areas.

FINDING A PRACTITIONER
- Ask your doctor. You may be able to get an NHS referral.
- Contact The Society of Teachers of the Alexander Technique.

WHAT'S INVOLVED
Lessons take place on a one-to-one basis. Sessions usually last for 30–40 minutes; most people need 20–30 lessons. During the lesson, a teacher may ask you to demonstrate sitting, standing and moving, and will show you how to replace any bad habits with better ones.

You will be asked to practise between sessions to help you to adapt to new ways of moving.

CONTACT **The Society of Teachers of the Alexander Technique** 1st floor, Linton House, 39-51 Highgate Road, London NW5 1RS 0845 230 7828 (www.stat.org.uk)

Alkaloids

Alkaloids are drugs, mostly of plant origin, that contain nitrogen and are weakly alkaline. Many are used in medicine, including morphine, from the opium poppy; atropine, from the belladonna plant group; vinblastine, a vinca alkaloid; and quinine, from cinchona tree bark and used in the treatment of malaria.
SEE ALSO **Drugs, medicinal**

Alkalosis

Alkalosis is a disturbance in the body's acid/alkali balance that results in the blood and body fluids becoming too alkaline. The acid/alkali balance is regulated by the lungs and kidneys. There are various types of alkalosis, each with different causes. Symptoms include confusion, muscle twitches, tremor in the hands, nausea and vomiting, lightheadedness, and numbness or tingling. Treatment consists of correcting the underlying cause, but in severe cases a saline (salt) drip or other treatment may be needed.
SEE ALSO **Acidosis; Adrenal glands and disorders**

Allergic rhinitis

Allergic rhinitis is an inflammation of the moist lining (mucous membrane) of the nose, caused by a reaction to an irritant. This results in attacks of sneezing, nasal discharge or a blocked nose. Excess mucus may also drip into the throat and cause soreness and coughing.

An attack typically lasts for more than an hour. In hay fever (seasonal allergic rhinitis), the problem is limited to a particular time of year; in perennial allergic rhinitis the nasal problems occur throughout the year.

Hay fever

Hay fever is neither caused by hay nor linked with fever. It is the most common of all allergic diseases, affecting 2–10 per cent of people worldwide. Many sufferers will have developed

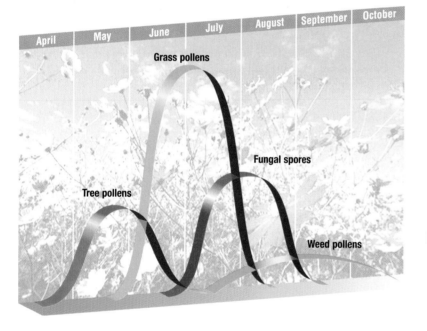

some symptoms by the age of ten, but there is an increase in the onset in adulthood. It rarely starts in people aged over 60. Annual hay fever attacks vary in severity and can recur for 10–15 years, after which they become less troublesome and eventually cease (see also **Hay fever**).

The trigger (allergen) that causes the allergic reaction is pollen from grass, trees, shrubs, weeds or flowers, and spores from moulds and fungi. Pollen counts (the percentage of pollen grains that can be measured in a cubic metre of air) are highest during spring and summer, this is when the plants and grasses that rely on the wind for cross-pollination release their pollen into the air. Twenty per cent of young people in the UK suffer the symptoms of hay fever in the peak months of June and July.

▲ **Pollen calendar**
Sufferers benefit if they keep track of times at which pollen levels put them most at risk of allergic reactions. The graph indicates in which months the different pollens and spores are most common.

In the pollen calendar graph:
April, May, June, July, August, September, October
Grass pollens
Fungal spores
Tree pollens
Weed pollens

TREATMENT

To reduce exposure to pollen, drive with the car windows closed, keep your bedroom window shut at night, and avoid walking in the countryside, particularly in the late afternoon when pollen falls to ground level.

Over-the-counter **antihistamines** are the most common treatment for rhinitis. They are effective against sneezing, less so against a runny nose (rhinorrhoea). At one time antihistamines tended to cause drowsiness but modern, non-sedative forms of the drug can be used safely when driving.

Over-the-counter **decongestants** such as pseudoephedrine hydrochloride give relief from nasal discharge and blockage but should only be used for a few days. After longer periods, stopping the drug will cause a rebound swelling of the nasal passages.

Small doses of **corticosteroids** (prescription drugs administered as a nasal spray or drops) are also an effective treatment for rhinitis. They work especially well when combined with a non-sedative antihistamine. When symptoms are particularly severe and in times of stress a short course of **steroids** may be justified.

It is also possible for sufferers to receive injections of prepared pollens to desensitize them, but this method is rarely used because it occasionally causes severe allergic reactions and even death in hypersensitive people. If desensitization is considered, skin tests are needed beforehand to decide on the appropriate preparation of pollens.

Perennial allergic rhinitis

Year-round nasal problems are caused by allergens such as house dust mites, feathers and animal fur, or by allergy to certain foods or to drugs such as aspirin. Symptoms are similar to hay fever. Nasal congestion is common and can lead to blockage of the Eustachian tube. This prevents effective drainage of the middle ear and can cause hearing problems, especially in children. The main complications of prolonged allergic rhinitis are sinus infections (**sinusitis**) and growths inside the nose (nasal polyps).

TREATMENT

When specific allergens can be identified, the treatment is broadly the same as for hay fever. Corticosteroid nasal sprays and drops are an effective treatment. Decongestant nose drops or sprays should not be used for more than a few days (as mentioned above).

SEE ALSO *Hay fever; Nose and problems*

CONTACT **The National Pollen Research Unit** issues a daily pollen guide (01905) 855 223 (www.pollenforecast.org.uk)

Allergies

Severe allergic reactions can leave the victim weak and nauseous or gasping for air. Some reactions can even be fatal. People with allergies must learn to identify and avoid the triggers that bring on their attacks.

If you have an allergy, your body is sensitive to – and therefore reacts to – one or more of the many substances to which people are exposed in everyday life. Substances that cause the body to react are called allergens; they include animal hair, pollen, house dust mites and foods such as eggs and shellfish. Allergens may be eaten, inhaled, touched or, in the case of an insect sting, injected under the skin. The allergic reaction often follows quickly. A wide variety of apparently unrelated ailments – such as **asthma, hay fever, eczema**, contact **dermatitis, nettlerash** (urticaria or hives) – are usually caused by allergies.

When allergens invade the body of an allergic person, the body defends itself by producing antibodies – proteins designed to neutralize the allergens. It is the subsequent reaction between antibody and allergen inside the body that produces the sufferer's allergic ailments.

Some people are allergic to the metallic element nickel, and come out in a rash on contact with it. It is present in some jewellery and coins.

HOW THE BODY RESPONDS TO ALLERGENS

People prone to allergies produce more of a particular type of immunoglobulin, called IgE. IgE forms after the initial contact with an allergen, and becomes attached to cells in the tissues, known as mast cells. When the body encounters the same allergen again it may react with the IgE, causing the mast cells to release a number of chemicals, including histamine. These chemicals cause swelling and inflammation in the surrounding tissues and give rise to various allergic symptoms, depending on which part of the body is affected.

NON-ALLERGIC REACTIONS

Around 10 per cent of hospital patients who are prescribed **penicillin** show a skin rash, but this is not a true allergy and is not serious; however, 0.1–0.4 per cent of those patients react with severe allergic symptoms including Anaphylactic shock (see page 92). A skin test that determines whether or not an individual is sensitive to penicillin is available.

Sometimes allergy-like symptoms are caused by something other than an allergy. For example, histamine can be released in response to an injury, such as a skin graze or damage to the delicate lining of the air passages when certain chemical fumes are inhaled. In these cases, the release of histamine creates allergy-like symptoms although no allergen is involved. Likewise, in susceptible

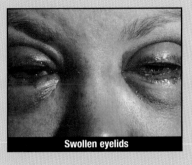
Swollen eyelids

▲ **Allergic reaction**
Swollen eyelids are often a symptom of hay fever. Try not to rub your eyelids. Bathing them in a warm salt solution may help.

Foods that cause allergy-like symptoms

Foods that trigger the release of histamine and foods that contain histamine can provoke allergy-like symptoms in a reaction known as 'false food allergy' or histamine toxicity.

Foods that contain histamine
- Well-ripened cheeses such as mature Brie or Camembert
- Continental sausages
- Some types of fish, especially mackerel or tuna, if they were not kept at a low temperature before being canned or eaten
- Fermented foods, including vinegar and alcoholic drinks, especially red wine.

Foods that trigger histamine release
- Peanuts, beans, peas and lentils
- Fish
- Egg white
- Strawberries
- Tomatoes
- Pork
- Chocolate
- Alcohol
- Shellfish: prawns, shrimps, crabs and lobsters.

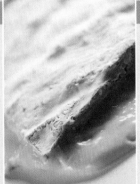
▲ **Histamine foods**
The histamine content of soft cheese increases as it ripens.

people, allergy-like symptoms can be caused by certain foods that trigger the release of histamine. Other foods can cause similar symptoms because they actually contain histamine (see Foods that cause allergy-like symptoms, page 91).

Food intolerance is another reaction that is sometimes confused with food allergy. In food intolerance a number of symptoms, such as headaches, emotional changes, painful joints and muscles, and fluid retention, appear to be caused by eating certain foods.

In such cases there is no hard evidence that the immune system is involved. Doctors do not consider the reaction to be a true allergy, but they find that temporary exclusion of certain foods can relieve symptoms.

WHY ARE ALLERGIES SO COMMON?

Allergies were once rare, but today they affect one-fifth of the population in the developed world. The reason for this increase is not really known, but there are many possible causes.
■ Early exposure, even before birth, to foods that commonly cause an allergic reaction, such as eggs, cow's milk, peanuts and sesame seeds.
■ Increased exposure to the droppings of house dust mites and to mould spores, because houses are generally more heavily carpeted, warmer and better insulated than in the past (see also **Asthma**).
■ Overprotection of young children from unclean environments and natural infections, which may

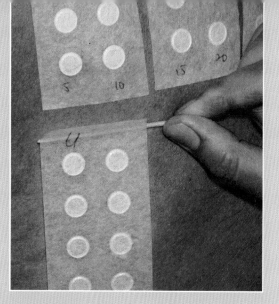

◀ **Patch testing**
Anyone with a contact skin allergy can undergo a test to identify possible allergens. A piece of non-allergenic tape holds samples of the allergens in place for 48 hours, after which the skin is inspected for the redness or swelling that would indicate allergy.

possibly alter the way in which the immune system matures.
■ Increased exposure to industrial pollution and man-made chemicals, including pesticides, insecticides and food additives.
■ Diets that contain too few vitamins and minerals.

TESTING FOR ALLERGIES

Skin and blood tests can help doctors to identify the allergens that may be causing allergic reactions. In a skin-prick test, small amounts of suspected allergens are introduced just under the skin. A weal will develop in the area within a few minutes if the person is allergic to the tested substance. (See **Blood and disorders; Patch test**.)

Factfile

Anaphylactic shock

Anaphylactic shock (or anaphylaxis) is an extreme allergic reaction. It can occur within minutes of contact with an allergen or be delayed for several hours. In rare cases it results in death.

Symptoms

■ Itching and swelling around the face and inside the mouth, including the tongue and throat.

■ Difficulty in breathing, together with wheezing, sneezing and a runny nose.

■ Flushed skin and nettle rash (urticaria or hives).

■ Rapid heartbeat and feelings of weakness.

■ Stomach cramps, diarrhoea or nausea.

■ Collapse and loss of consciousness may follow.

What to do if you are at risk

■ If you are at risk of anaphylaxis, carry adrenaline with you at all times and become familiar with how to inject it into your muscles. Label the packs so that someone else can administer the adrenaline in an emergency.

Pre-assembled syringes with adult or child doses are the easiest to cope with.

How to help a victim of anaphylactic shock

■ If the victim has had a previous attack and carries antihistamine medication and an adrenaline injection, these should be given as soon as possible. Adrenaline injections may need to be repeated once or twice at 15-minute intervals. Unless an adrenalin auto-injector is used, the adrenaline should be injected slowly for those with a heart condition, high blood pressure or diabetes.

■ Always send for medical help or an ambulance.

■ Loosen clothing at the neck and around the waist, help the victim to lie down and raise the legs and feet a little if you can. Keep the airway open.

■ If the cause was a bee sting, flick out any remaining sting with your fingernail: avoid squeezing it, because a bee sting contains venom.

■ Anaphylactic shock may develop over the course of a few hours: consult your doctor if the above symptoms occur within a couple of hours of a meal.

LIVING WITH ALLERGIES

These strategies will help you to avoid allergic reactions as far as possible while living a full life.
■ Try to identify your allergic triggers. Because these triggers are individual to you, you can minimize the effort needed to avoid allergic attacks if you have a precise idea of what causes your symptoms.
■ Always carry your medication with you, especially if you have asthma, food allergies or are allergic to insect stings.
■ Eat a well-balanced diet, including two to four fruits and three to five vegetables each day.

ALLERGIES IN CHILDREN

Children have less developed immune systems than adults, which makes them vulnerable to irritants in the environment such as pollen and the droppings of house dust mites. Asthma, eczema and hay fever are the commonest types of allergy in children and may be inherited. As children's immune systems develop, many childhood allergies disappear and most have gone by the time a person reaches adulthood. One common exception is a nut allergy, which usually proves to be a lifelong affliction.

ALLERGY MEDICINES

Several types of conventional medication can be used to relieve allergies; treatment will vary depending on the type and severity of the allergy.

Antihistamine preparations block the action of histamine, while mast-cell stabilizing drugs prevent the release of histamine. Other treaments include **corticosteroids**, which suppress the allergic reactions, adrenaline injections, which are used for anaphylaxis (see box, far left) and desensitization, which involves injecting small doses of the allergen.

COMPLEMENTARY THERAPIES

Many complementary therapists recommend stress management, which can improve the action of the immune system. Changes in diet can also help. **Herbal** or **dietary supplements** and **homeopathic medicines** can benefit some allergy sufferers, too. Homeopaths may use remedies made from the allergen that triggers a patient's symptoms, if this is known.

Complementary therapists also use various diagnostic tests: there is little or no scientific support for these tests, but they seem to help some people identify the cause of their allergy. They include pulse tests (checking if the pulse rate is altered by eating a suspect food); the sublingual drop test (which means observing reactions to the application of a suspect substance under the tongue); and an elimination diet (in which the effects of reintroducing suspect foods after they have been excluded are observed).

SEE ALSO *Immune system*

CONTACT **British Allergy Foundation**
30 Bellegrove Road, Welling,
Kent DA16 3PY; helpline (020) 8303 8583
9am–5pm Mon–Fri
(www.allergyfoundation.com)
**British Society for Allergy,
Environmental and Nutritional
Medicine** PO Box 7, Knighton, Powys
LD8 2WF (01547) 550 380
(www.jnem.demon.co.uk)

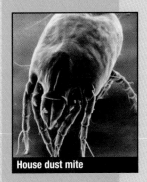

When inhaled, cat dander (tiny flakes of dried saliva found on cat skin and hair) and the droppings of house dust mites are triggers for asthma attacks and other allergies.

House dust mite

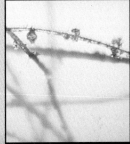

Dander on cat hair

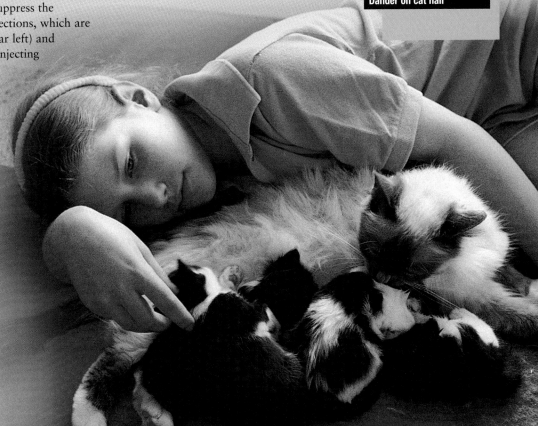

▶ Cat allergy
People who are allergic to cat dander must avoid contact with cats and kittens and be careful not to touch their face or eyes without first washing their hands.

Alopecia

Alopecia is the medical word for **baldness**. The most common form is male pattern baldness, or androgenic alopecia, which usually affects older men. The term 'alopecia' is also used to refer to hair-loss conditions in which hair follicles stop growing either on a small patch of skin, in one region of the body, or sometimes all over the body. In alopecia areata, for example, hair is lost in patches, usually on the scalp. About 15 per cent of people in the UK are affected at some time by one of these conditions.

CAUSES

Apart from male pattern baldness, which is hereditary, the various forms of alopecia are thought to be caused by an overactive immune system attacking the hair follicles. **Stress** plays a major role in triggering hair loss because it reduces blood supply to the scalp; it also seems to increase production of oily secretions by the sebaceous glands connected to each hair follicle.

Occasionally the condition is linked to iron-deficiency **anaemia** or to problems with the **thyroid** gland. Alopecia following illness or pregnancy rarely lasts more than six months.

TREATMENT

There is no cure for male pattern baldness. In alopecia areata, a doctor may carry out blood tests to check if the cause is a lack of iron or an inefficient thyroid gland. Treatments such as **corticosteroid** injections are not fully effective, although the drug minoxidil may stop hair loss.

Complementary and other therapies

■ Homeopathic remedies may help. For alopecia linked with emotional trauma, try a 30c dose of Natrum muriaticum (Nat. mur.) once a week.
■ Massaging the scalp helps to encourage blood flow and to stimulate hair follicles.
■ Cosmetic hair design involves weaving artificial hair fibres into your own hair or onto a fine mesh net to disguise areas of hair loss.

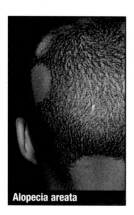

▼ Irregular hair loss
Hair that comes out in patches could be due to iron deficiency or thyroid problems and should be checked by a doctor.

Alopecia areata

Main types of alopecia

There are various forms of alopecia; hair may be lost from just the scalp or the entire body.

Androgenic alopecia (male pattern baldness)
Hair loss occurs over the scalp; the condition mostly affects older men.

Alopecia areata Hair is lost in patches, usually on the scalp.

Alopecia totalis Total loss of scalp hair.

Alopecia universalis Loss of hair over the entire body, including eyebrows and eyelashes.

OUTLOOK

In many cases, alopecia areata improves over time. In half of all cases, the hair follicles start to recover within a year, and the hair begins to grow back. Four out of five sufferers from alopecia areata regrow their hair within five years, but some always retain a small bald area.

In around one in ten people affected by alopecia areata, the condition progressively worsens. Occasionally, the affected area may grow larger. In rare circumstances, patchy hair loss or general thinning eventually extends all over the scalp to produce alopecia totalis.

Altitude sickness

Altitude sickness, also called mountain sickness, affects people such as climbers and pilots in unpressurized aircraft who are not adapted to living at high altitudes. It can also affect tourists and travellers visiting high altitudes.

People are vulnerable to altitude sickness when they ascend rapidly to heights of more than 2400–3000m (8000–10,000ft) above sea level. Air pressure falls with altitude, so at progressively higher altitudes each breath of air contains less oxygen. The levels of oxygen in the blood fall, so that the tissues are deprived of this vital nutrient. To compensate, the heart rate increases, speeding blood flow through the lungs and brain. The lungs can become saturated with water, or fluid may leak into the brain, which can be fatal. Exertion may strain the heart, causing a heart attack.

Gradual ascent is the best way to avoid the problem. Children, elderly people and anyone with lung or heart disease should consult a doctor before travelling to high altitudes.

SYMPTOMS

Symptoms may appear between 8 and 48 hours after rapid ascent to high altitude. They include:
■ feverishness and severe headache;
■ dizziness and unsteadiness;
■ nausea and vomiting;
■ mental slowness and confusion;
■ muscular lethargy and paralysis;
■ tightness in the chest and breathlessness;
■ loss of appetite and weight;
■ insomnia;
■ impaired vision and speech;
■ euphoria and hallucinations.

TREATMENT

Relatively mild symptoms subside after a few days of rest. People with severe symptoms must descend rapidly to lower altitudes and report to a doctor at once. Breathing in oxygen from a pressurized supply may relieve the effects of fluid in the lungs or brain.

Alzheimer's disease

Although Alzheimer's cannot be cured, much can be done to make life easier for people with the condition. New drugs work best in the early stages of the disease, so an early diagnosis is becoming more important.

Alzheimer's disease is the most common cause of **dementia** – a group of symptoms that includes confusion, memory loss, mood changes and speech problems. About 500,000 people in the UK suffer from Alzheimer's, and most are elderly. The condition affects about one in 20 people over the age of 65 and one in five over the age of 80.

A rarer form of Alzheimer's, which tends to run in families, can occur at a much younger age, affecting people in their 30s or 40s. Commoner forms of the disease also appear to have genetic links, but there is no single genetic mutation as occurs with true genetic disorders such as cystic fibrosis.

WHO IS AT RISK?

Research into Alzheimer's disease has identified a 'susceptibility gene' called apolipoprotein E (ApoE). It has been demonstrated that the risk of developing the disease in old age depends at least in part on the configuration of ApoE genes that an individual has inherited.

◀ **Helping hand**
The confusion and disorientation caused by Alzheimer's mean that people with the disease need increasing help with daily activities such as feeding and dressing. In the later stages, full-time residential care becomes necessary.

A wide variety of environmental factors have also been investigated as possible triggers of the disease, especially in genetically susceptible individuals. ApoE plays a role in cholesterol metabolism and heart disease – and people with high cholesterol or high blood pressure, and those who smoke, are all known to have an increased risk of developing Alzheimer's disease. Those who have suffered head or whiplash injuries also seem to be at risk. However, research has failed to support the idea that exposure to aluminium increases the risk of Alzheimer's.

CHARACTERISTICS OF THE DISEASE

Many people complain of poor memory as they grow older, but those with Alzheimer's disease become increasingly forgetful and confused, and this may make them frustrated, angry or frightened. As often happens in elderly people, old memories may remain intact whereas recent events are soon forgotten. People with Alzheimer's also have difficulty finding appropriate words and solving basic problems, and they may show signs of language impairment, such as rambling speech, long pauses and repetition. They are likely to become disorientated and perhaps get lost in familiar places.

As the disease progresses, everyday activities such as dressing, shopping and cooking become increasingly difficult. People with Alzheimer's find it harder and harder to communicate. They may become depressed and lose interest in the outside world; they are likely to give up interests and hobbies and become indifferent to social conventions and the opinions of others.

Alzheimer's disease is not the only reason why elderly people become confused. Circulatory problems, strokes and the side effects of certain medicines can also cause dementia-like symptoms. It is therefore important to seek medical help for anyone who is becoming confused or forgetful, so that any problems can be swiftly assessed and treated by an expert.

WHAT IS ALZHEIMER'S DISEASE?

First described in 1907 by Alois Alzheimer, a German neurologist, the disease attacks the thinking parts of the brain, including the

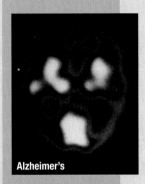

Alzheimer's

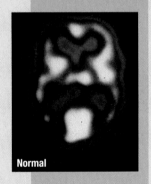

Normal

hippocampus, one of the memory centres. Nerve fibres become tangled (neurofibrillary tangles) and clumps of abnormal protein (neuritic plaques) appear. Cells are destroyed and the brain shrinks. Some of these changes – the shrinkage of brain tissue and enlargement of the fluid-filled ventricles at the centre of the brain – are visible on brain scans. But tangles and plaques are visible under the microscope only when cells from the brain of someone with Alzheimer's is examined after death.

TREATMENT

The nerve damage seen in Alzheimer's disease includes a fall in the nerve transmitter acetylcholine, one of a group of chemicals in the brain that carries messages from one nerve to the next. Drugs currently used to treat the disease are aimed at restoring acetylcholine levels. They include donepezil (brand name Aricept), memantine (Ebixa), rivastigmine (Exelon) and galantamine (Reminyl). These drugs, if taken in the early stages of the illness, can slow or halt the deterioration of some patients for several months. They seem to improve the quality of life of people with Alzheimer's, enabling them to feel more alert and more willing to take part in social activities.

Complementary treatments such as music therapy and aromatherapy may be helpful to some people.

A POSSIBLE VACCINE

Future treatments are likely to be targeted at two proteins that seem to play key roles in the development of neurofibrillary tangles and neuritic plaques. The first protein, called tau, normally holds nerve fibres together so that they can carry messages efficiently. In Alzheimer's, a chemical change in tau makes it break away from nerve fibres, which then become tangled. Researchers are therefore looking for drugs that can stabilize tau so that nerve fibres stay neat and tidy. The second protein, called beta amyloid, forms the core of neuritic plaques. Some types of beta amyloid are more harmful than others, and scientists are trying to design drugs that will block production of the harmful varieties.

Trials are also underway to test a vaccine that uses one type of the beta amyloid protein to try to trigger a protective immune response. If this is strong enough, it may help to prevent formation of neuritic plaques.

SEE ALSO *Brain and nervous system; Genetics and genetic disorders.*

CONTACT **Alzheimer's Society** Gordon House, 10 Greencoat Place, London SW1P 1PH; helpline 0845 300 0336 (www.alzheimers.org.uk) Help for people with Alzheimer's, as well as for their families and their carers.
Mind 15–19 Broadway, London E15 4BQ; Mind*info*line 0845 766 0163 9.15am–5.15pm Mon–Fri (www.mind.org.uk). Campaigns for improved mental health services in England and Wales; publishes booklets and leaflets.
Carers UK Ruth Pitter House, 20–25 Glasshouse Yard, London EC1A 4JT; helpline 0808 808 7777 10am–12pm and 2pm-4pm Wed & Thurs. Advice and support for carers of the ill, frail or disabled.
Alzheimer's Research Trust Livanos House, Granhams Road, Cambridge CB2 5LQ (01223) 843 899 (www.alzheimers-research.org.uk) Researching causes, treatment and prevention.

Guidelines for carers

Carers of people with Alzheimer's can do much to help them to lead lives that are as normal as possible, at least in the disease's early stages.

As a person's mental function deteriorates, full-time residential care is likely to be needed. But thousands of people with early Alzheimer's disease are cared for at home by family and friends. This can be emotionally and physically exhausting for the carers. Availability of support and respite care varies from area to area – local branches of national charities and support groups should be able to advise.

People with Alzheimer's disease often have to make difficult financial and healthcare decisions, and it helps if carers are as honest as possible about what is happening.

There are a number of practical ways to help people with Alzheimer's disease to cope with daily life.

■ Draw up lists of things than need to be done during the day such as washing, getting dressed and preparing food.

■ Label appliances and places where things are kept as a memory aid.

■ Reduce potential hazards – check the safety of cookers and fires, for example.

■ Arrange for home visits by workers from social and other services.

■ Try memory therapy. For example, sit down with the person to look at old photographs and discuss notable family events.

Amblyopia

Amblyopia is a disorder in which the sharpness of vision is impaired. It is usually associated with a problem that prevents normal use of the eye in early childhood, such as an uncorrected squint, congenital cataract or **astigmatism**. As a result, a clear image does not form on the retina and the normal appreciation of vision in the brain does not develop properly.

In some cases, amblyopia is due to optic nerve damage caused by excessive alcohol intake or tobacco use, poor diet or drugs. The condition is usually successfully treated only in children under eight years old. When caused by a squint, a patch is placed over the good eye, forcing the other eye to function properly. Congenital cataracts are removed by surgery. Glasses can help to correct severe focusing problems.
SEE ALSO *Eye and problems*

Amenorrhoea

Amenorrhoea is the absence of menstrual periods. Apart from pregnancy, causes include hormonal problems, being underweight, **stress** and **anaemia**. Periods are often absent in top athletes and in people with **anorexia nervosa**.

The term 'primary amenorrhoea' is used to describe the condition in which periods have never started, whereas 'secondary amenorrhoea' indicates that a woman has had periods but that they have stopped. Neither is the same thing as oligomenorrhoea (very light periods).
SEE ALSO *Menstruation*

Amino acids

Amino acids are the building blocks of proteins. There are more than 20 amino acids, most of which can be synthesized by the body. Others cannot be made in the body and must form part of the diet – these are called essential amino acids. Proteins in food are broken down in the body into their constituent amino acids and used to make new proteins as required.

People born with the rare genetic condition phenylketonuria are unable fully to break down the amino acid phenylalamine. They must eat a special diet for life to avoid dangerous effects.

Amnesia

Amnesia is a loss of memory, either partial or total, caused by disease or injury to the brain, or sometimes by drugs or psychological trauma.

In retrograde amnesia, memory about facts or events before the trauma is lost. In anterograde amnesia, memory about events after the trauma is affected. Some people experience both types.

Someone suffering from amnesia caused by a viral infection may find it difficult to identify common objects or remember the meaning of ordinary words.

DURATION
Memory may return within minutes or hours, or more gradually. It may return only when the underlying condition has cleared up. In cases of severe brain injury or progressive diseases, amnesia can worsen or become permanent.

SYMPTOMS
Anterograde amnesia varies from a total lack of recall of events just after an accident to minor difficulty in retaining day-to-day information. It may involve a more serious loss of memory, perhaps leading to permanent disorientation.

Retrograde amnesia may vary from the inability to remember the period just before an accident or the onset of disease to difficulty in remembering minor details. Some affected people are unable to recall anything that has happened in the past 20 years.

CAUSES
Amnesia has many possible causes:
- head injury;
- emotional shock;
- **Alzheimer's disease** and **dementia**;
- **meningitis**, **encephalitis** and other viral infections;
- brain tumours, brain haemorrhages (see **Brain and nervous system**) and **strokes**;
- heavy drinking or malnourishment.

TREATMENT
If any symptoms of amnesia are noticed after an injury or shock, or if you suffer from repeated bouts of amnesia, seek medical advice.

What a doctor may do
Depending on the suspected source of the amnesia, a doctor may do one of the following.
- Test you for infections or other diseases, and possibly arrange for you to have a brain scan or to see a neurologist or neuropsychologist.
- If the amnesia is due to an emotional shock, refer you for psychiatric help.
- In the case of malnourishment, administer thiamin (vitamin B_1) injections.

Complementary therapies
Treatments such as **massage** and **acupuncture** may improve relaxation and thereby reduce the level of stress.

PREVENTION
Amnesia due to trauma or disease is not preventable. Memory training and continued intellectual stimulation can help to keep memory sharp well into old age.

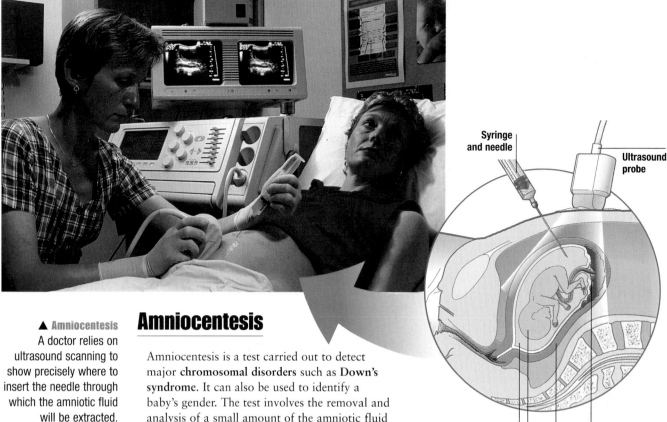

Syringe and needle

Ultrasound probe

Amniotic fluid
Fetus
Womb
Placenta

▲ **Amniocentesis**
A doctor relies on ultrasound scanning to show precisely where to insert the needle through which the amniotic fluid will be extracted.

Amniocentesis

Amniocentesis is a test carried out to detect major **chromosomal disorders** such as **Down's syndrome**. It can also be used to identify a baby's gender. The test involves the removal and analysis of a small amount of the amniotic fluid surrounding a developing baby in the womb. Although a woman may choose to undergo an amniocentesis in order to prepare for the possibility that she and her partner will have an affected baby, the procedure also means that she can choose to terminate the pregnancy if the test results are positive. Hospitals routinely offer amniocentesis to a pregnant woman in any of the following circumstances.

■ She has previously had a child affected by a chromosomal abnormality.

■ She has had a pregnancy terminated for this reason before.

■ She is aged over 35, since the risk increases sharply after this age.

■ Previous blood tests or scans have raised cause for concern.

WHAT'S INVOLVED

The usual time for performing an amniocentesis is 13–15 weeks after conception, but at some clinical research centres it can be carried out as early as 11 weeks.

Guided by an **ultrasound** scan, a specialist passes a fine needle through the mother's abdominal wall and into her womb, removing the equivalent of one to four teaspoons of the amniotic fluid surrounding the baby.

Women vary in the amount of discomfort they feel – there is usually the option of having a local **anaesthetic** to numb the area around the point of entry. After the test, it is advisable for the woman to rest for the remainder of the day.

Stray fetal cells found in the fluid sample are analysed in a laboratory. The results arrive three to five weeks later and are 99 per cent accurate.

RISKS

The test carries a risk of up to one per cent of causing a miscarriage, and there is also a one per cent possibility that it may cause severe breathing problems for the baby at birth.

SEE ALSO *Pregnancy and problems; Pregnancy, termination of*

CONTACT **The National Childbirth Trust**
Alexandra House, Oldham Terrace, Acton, London W3 6NH; helpline 0870 444 8707 (www.nctpregnancyandbabycare.com)
Antenatal Results and Choices 73–75 Charlotte Street, London W1T 4PN; helpline (020) 7631 0285 (www.arc-uk.org) Support for parents on all aspects of fetal tests.

Amoebiasis

Amoebiasis is a parasitic infection found mostly in tropical countries. It is usually caught by eating raw food such as unpeeled fruit or vegetables contaminated by human faeces. Cooking destroys *Entamoeba histolytica*, the parasite that causes amoebiasis.

Symptoms include moderate **diarrhoea**, and abdominal cramps. Amoebic dysentery is when symptoms become more acute and there is severe diarrhoea containing blood and mucus.

SEE ALSO *Parasites and parasitic diseases; Travel and health; Tropical diseases*

Amputation

Amputation is the surgical removal of part or all of a limb or other body appendage. It is usually performed to prevent the spread of infection or cancerous cells from diseased to healthy tissues, or to remove all or part of a limb that can no longer function, thus enabling an artificial limb (prosthesis) to be fitted.

WHO IT CAN HELP

■ People suffering from conditions such as **thrombosis** or peripheral vascular disease, in which the narrowing of the blood vessels in the legs and arms can cause the blood supply to be completely blocked, causing **gangrene**.

■ People with bone **cancer** or malignant melanoma (a type of skin cancer) who need the limb removed to prevent the disease from spreading.

■ People who have a limb damaged irreparably through injury or frostbite.

WHAT'S INVOLVED

A specialist surgeon uses a combination of physical examination and **X-ray** techniques such as angiography to decide where the amputation should be made.

The operation involves skin and muscle being cut lower than the bone in order to create a flap to cover the stump. To minimize pain from the pressure that occurs when the patient uses an artificial limb, the nerves above the stump are severed.

After the operation, it may take several weeks for the wound to heal. Sometimes people experience **phantom limb pain**, in which the brain misinterprets signals from the nerves at the site of amputation so that the person feels a sensation where the limb used to be.

Amyloid disease

Amyloid disease is a rare disorder in which amyloid, a wax-like protein, builds up in tissues and organs including the heart, liver, kidneys and spleen. It is usually a complication of another disease such as rheumatoid **arthritis, tuberculosis, Hodgkin's disease, ulcerative colitis** and bone marrow **cancer**. The affected organs often become enlarged. If the heart is affected, there may be an irregular heartbeat or heart failure; if the stomach is affected, ulceration and diarrhoea may develop. Waxy bumps sometimes appear on the face, neck and groin. There is no treatment; when amyloid disease is secondary, it may be reversed if the underlying illness is treated.

Anabolic steroids

Anabolic steroids are synthetic hormones that promote tissue growth; most are synthetic forms of male hormones related to **testosterone**. They are sometimes used to halt weight loss in elderly or seriously ill patients. They may also be used to boost blood cell production in the bone marrow of patients with blood disorders, or to treat post menopausal **osteoporosis**.

Since they act in the body to stimulate protein synthesis, thereby increasing muscle strength and bulk, anabolic **steroids may be abused by athletes who a**re willing to endanger their health in the quest for sporting success. Long-term use can lead to serious side effects such as liver cancer and aggressive behaviour.

SEE ALSO *Drugs, medicinal*

Women who take anabolic steroids may notice masculinizing effects such as an increase in body hair or a deepening of the voice.

Artificial limbs

Ready-made prostheses are available, but the best are those that have been specifically tailored to a patient's needs.

Artificial limbs need to be comfortable, light and unobtrusive, and to function as effectively as possible. Some limbs, especially artificial hands and arms, are electronically controlled – circuitry in the limb responds to nerve impulses in the stump. Whole artificial legs are attached using straps; for amputations below the knee, newer kinds of prostheses use suction rather than traps, making them easier to put on and take off. Advances in cosmetic skin and silicone technology have improved the realistic appearance of all types of artificial limb. In addition, recent developments with microcomputers have produced legs and knee joints that can adapt to a person's natural walking pattern.

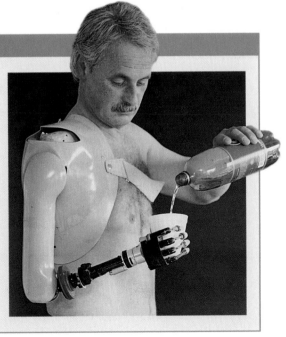

Anaemia

Anaemia is a condition in which the quantity of oxygen-carrying haemoglobin in the **blood** is below normal. It is the most widespread of all blood disorders, and can occur in many forms, principally iron-deficiency, megaloblastic, sickle cell, haemolytic and aplastic anaemias.

SYMPTOMS

These symptoms are common to all types of anaemia:

- fatigue;
- shortness of breath;
- dizziness and disturbed vision;
- headaches and insomnia;
- palpitations;
- pale skin;
- loss of appetite and indigestion;
- in severe cases, swelling of the ankles;
- in older people, chest pain.

Iron-deficiency anaemia

Iron-deficiency anaemia is the most common form of the disorder. It is caused by a shortage of iron in the blood. This prevents the bone marrow from making enough haemoglobin, the oxygen-carrying pigment in red blood cells – with the result that the body does not get enough oxygen. The condition persists until treated unless the cause is temporary, in which case the body will slowly build up the deficit.

Depending on the cause, the condition could be corrected within three to six weeks of starting treatment. The person may then need to take an iron supplement for six months.

SYMPTOMS

In addition to the symptoms common to all types of anaemia, people with the iron-deficient form suffer from dry, brittle nails and a sore tongue and mouth. In very severe cases, heart failure and **oedema** may occur.

CAUSES

- Loss of blood due to heavy periods (see **Menstruation and problems**).
- Excessive bleeding resulting from an accident or due to surgery.
- A diet deficient in iron.
- **Pregnancy**, which increases the body's need for iron.
- Poor absorption of iron from the diet, usually due to surgical removal of part of the stomach, or to **coeliac disease**.
- Diseases in which there is persistent bleeding, such as **gastritis**, peptic ulcer, bowel disorders including bowel cancer, haemorrhoids (piles) and urinary tract infections.

TREATMENT

Seek medical advice if any of the above symptoms develop.

What a doctor may do

- Carry out tests to measure the level of iron in the blood and the number of red blood cells.
- Investigate any underlying cause of the symptoms, for example, using **endoscopy** or barium X-rays (see **Barium investigations**) to check for digestive tract disorders.
- If the diagnosis is confirmed, prescribe iron-supplement tablets, or occasionally give iron by injection.
- Prescribe drugs that control excessive menstrual bleeding.

What you can do

Eat plenty of iron-rich foods such as lean meat, green vegetables, wholemeal bread, pulses, eggs and dried fruits. Avoid drinking tea with meals, since this can inhibit the absorption of iron from food.

Megaloblastic anaemia

This form of the disorder, also known as pernicious anaemia, results from a lack of either vitamin B_{12} or folic acid, which prevents the effective production of red blood cells in the bone marrow. The condition persists until treated.

Some surgery is known to cause a deficiency of vitamin B_{12}. Patients who have undergone such surgery can be given injection of vitamin B_{12} to counteract the problems.

With treatment, the outlook for recovery is good, but to prevent recurrence you may need to have B_{12} injections or take folic acid tablets for an indefinite period.

SYMPTOMS

Apart from the symptoms common to all types of anaemia, people with megaloblastic anaemia may have persistent diarrhoea, tingling in the fingers and toes, and a sore tongue. Some may also develop jaundice, which produces a yellowish tinge in the eyes and the skin.

If treatment does not begin within six months of the onset of symptoms, the central nervous system may be irreversibly damaged. Other complications include heart failure, stomach cancer and degeneration of the spinal cord.

CAUSES

- An inability to absorb vitamin B_{12} – often as the result of an **autoimmune disease**. This condition is usually hereditary and is sometimes linked with **diabetes** or **myxoedema**.
- Folic acid deficiency.
- Removal of the small intestine, or the complete removal of the stomach.
- A vegan diet.
- Chronic alcohol abuse.
- Diseases that interfere with the absorption of foods by the body, such as **Crohn's disease** and **coeliac disease**.

TREATMENT

If you develop any of the symptoms described, seek medical advice.

What a doctor may do

- Take a blood sample to assess haemoglobin levels in the blood.
- Refer you to hospital for a bone marrow test.
- Carry out further tests if an underlying cause is suspected.
- Prescribe a course of vitamin B_{12} injections or folic acid tablets.

What you can do

- Eat foods rich in vitamin B_{12}, including meat, poultry, fish, cereals, dairy products and eggs, and foods rich in folic acid, including broccoli, spinach and wholemeal bread.
- During early pregnancy, take a course of folic acid supplements.

Sickle cell anaemia

Sickle cell anaemia is an inherited condition in which the red blood cells contain an abnormal type of haemoglobin. If, because of exertion or respiratory infection, the amount of oxygen in the blood is reduced, the abnormal haemoglobin causes the blood cells to deform into a crescent or sickle shape. These may block blood vessels, reducing blood flow to body tissues, and may be destroyed by the body's immune system. Sickle cell anaemia is found mainly in people of African and Afro-Caribbean descent.

Haemolytic anaemias

Haemolytic anaemias are a group of disorders in which red blood cells are produced at the normal rate but destroyed much faster than usual. The condition may be:

- due to an inherited defect;
- acquired later in life, through an **autoimmune disease**, for example;
- associated with other conditions such as **leukaemia** or **lupus**;
- due to an infectious disease such as **pneumonia** or **malaria**;
- caused by treatment with certain drugs.

TREATMENT

Possible treatments include:

- the removal of the spleen, the organ in which many of the red blood cells are destroyed;
- immunosuppressant drugs;
- other medication such as antimalarial drugs.

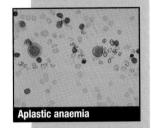
Aplastic anaemia

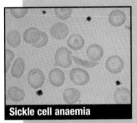
Megaloblastic anaemia

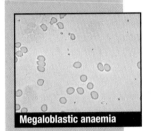
Sickle cell anaemia

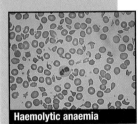
Haemolytic anaemia

Aplastic anaemia

Aplastic anaemia is a rare type of the disorder in which fewer red blood cells, white blood cells and platelets than normal are produced. It is caused by the bone marrow's inability to produce stem cells (the cells that form the basis of all cells in the body). Aplastic anaemia may be the result of a viral infection or an **autoimmune disease**, or it may be a side effect of various drugs or treatment for **cancer** such as **radiotherapy** or anticancer drugs. In many cases no cause can be found.

Symptoms can take the form of spontaneous bruising and repeated infections such as sore throats.

Treatment may involve a **blood transfusion**, drugs to stimulate blood cell production, or drugs to suppress the immune system. In severe cases of the disorder, a bone marrow transplant is usually needed.

Anaerobic exercise

Anaerobic exercise is any form of exercise that uses energy that is stored in muscles rather than relying on increased oxygen consumption.

Examples of anaerobic exercise include running 100 metres (108 yards), doing press-ups, weightlifting, and 'stop-go' racquet sports such as squash or tennis – all of which involve bursts of high-intensity activity.

Anaerobic training increases strength rather than stamina. It tones and firms muscles while adding to muscle bulk, and it also has positive effects on the body's insulin balance and blood pressure levels.

This form of exercise can be carried out for only limited periods of time, after which waste products build up in the muscles, forcing the person engaged in the exercise to stop and have a rest.

As a form of training, anaerobic exercise helps sports performance but does not aid cardiovascular fitness.

SEE ALSO *Aerobic exercise; Exercise and health*

Anaesthesia and anaesthetics

The development of anaesthetics in the 19th century was a key factor in the advance of modern surgery. Until then, surgery relied on alcohol and narcotics to subdue a patient, often with disastrous results. The drugs used today are easily administered and generally safe.

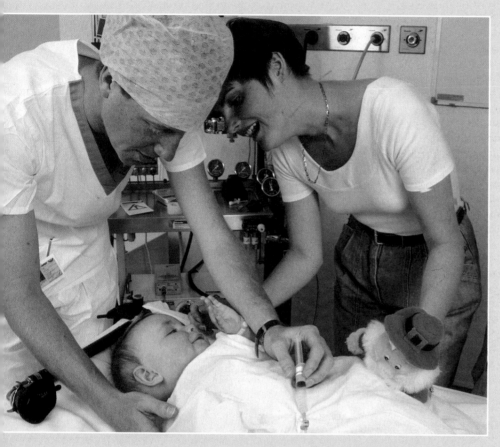

▲ **Parental support**
Parents are encouraged to accompany their children to the anaesthetic room and support them until they are asleep.

the patient and the surgical procedure involved. Patients are advised not to eat or drink for at least six hours before an operation to avoid the risk of vomiting and choking while under general anaesthesia. The anaesthetist monitors the patient throughout the operation, supervises recovery from the anaesthetic and advises on post-operative care, including pain management.

LOCAL ANAESTHESIA
In the case of a local or regional anaesthetic, drugs block all the sensation pathways in one part of the nervous system. This technique is often used in conjunction with general anaesthesia to ensure pain-free recovery. When only a local anaesthetic is used, patients remain conscious during the procedure; they feel no pain, although they may feel pulling or pressure in the area being treated.

Local anaesthetics are introduced directly into the appropriate part of the body or injected around the nerves supplying it. Their effect can be limited to, say, one finger or, in the case of dentistry, to a small part of the mouth.

A more specialized technique, known as an epidural, involves injecting an anaesthetic drug into the space around the spinal cord. This blocks off nerves serving the lower part of the body. Epidurals are well established as a form of pain relief during labour.

Local anaesthetic is usually given by injection, but sometimes an ointment, eyedrops, or a spray may be used. Local anaesthesia can also be induced by **acupuncture** and **hypnotherapy**.

RISKS AND COMPLICATIONS
Modern anaesthesia is now very safe, accounting for one death in 250,000. Always tell an anaesthetist if you are taking any medicines or suffer from any medical condition. Sometimes people experience nausea or vomiting after having an anaesthetic, but there are antisickness drugs to counter these after effects.

Anaesthesia means a loss of sensation. It may occur as the result of a disease, or follow trauma to a nerve. But the word is most often used to mean a loss of sensation induced by drugs. Anaesthesia allows surgical and other procedures to be carried out on patients without pain. There are two types of anaesthesia: general, and local or regional.

GENERAL ANAESTHESIA
In general anaesthesia, an anaesthetist (a doctor with at least six years' specialist training) gives drugs through a vein or by inhalation or, more often, a combination of both. The anaesthetist visits the patient before the operation to assess the individual's needs and answer any questions. Various drugs are used to produce a loss of consciousness and sensation; the anaesthetist chooses the most appropriate combination for

Analgesic drugs

Aspirin and other NSAIDs irritate the stomach lining and can cause bleeding and ulceration if taken in sufficient doses for a prolonged period.

Analgesics – also known as painkillers – are medicines that reduce pain without causing loss of consciousness and usually without affecting other sensations such as touch or temperature.

Mild analgesic drugs such as paracetamol, aspirin, ibuprofen and low-dose codeine (in combination with other drugs) are available over the counter for home treatment of ailments such as headache, toothache and period pain.

Aspirin, paracetamol and ibuprofen also act to reduce temperature and so can help to soothe fevers. Aspirin and ibuprofen are non-steroidal anti-inflammatory drugs (NSAIDs). These are useful for treating rheumatic conditions because they reduce inflammation. Some preparations sold over the counter are compound analgesics – they contain more than one painkilling drug.

Paracetamol is the analgesic drug of choice for children and can be used to reduce fever after immunization in babies. Use a children's formulation, such as Calpol.

Stronger painkilling drugs that may be prescribed by a doctor include more powerful NSAIDs (for alleviating conditions such as rheumatoid arthritis) and narcotic analgesics including morphine, pethidine and diamorphine (heroin), which are used to combat severe pain in conditions such as cancer. Narcotic analgesics should be used with care because they can produce dependency (see **Addictions; Drugs, medicinal; Painkillers**).

Analgesic drugs

The various analgesics have different modes of action and so have particular uses. Always follow the dosage guidelines on the packaging.

DRUG	REDUCES PAIN	REDUCES FEVER	REDUCES INFLAMMATION	ADDICTIVE POTENTIAL
Aspirin	✔	✔	✔	
Codeine	✔			✔
Paracetamol	✔	✔		
Co-codaprin (codeine and aspirin)	✔	✔	✔	✔
Co-codamol (codeine and paracetamol)	✔			✔
Other NSAIDs (including ibuprofen)	✔	✔	✔	✔

Anaphylactic shock

Anaphylactic shock is a rare but potentially life-threatening allergic reaction in which the body produces a massive amount of histamine. Symptoms include wheezing and a raised rash. Possible triggers are insect bites and stings, some drugs and foods such as peanuts. In the event of such an attack, medical attention should be sought immediately, and adrenaline injections administered if available.
SEE ALSO *Allergies*

Androgens

Male sex hormones, mainly testosterone, are known collectively as androgens. Those produced in the body are responsible for promoting signs of masculinity at puberty, such as the development of the sex organs, the growth of hair on the face and body, and the deepening of the voice. They are made mainly in the testes, but small amounts are also produced in the adrenal glands.

Women normally produce small amounts of androgens in the ovaries; if too much is made, unwanted effects can occur, including growth of hair in the beard area.

Synthetic androgens are manufactured for use as drugs to treat conditions such as delayed puberty, and may also be useful in the treatment of diseases such as breast cancer.

Anencephaly

Anencephaly is a severe fetal abnormality in which the neural tube (which forms the brain and spinal cord) fails to develop in the womb. It occurs in one in 1000 pregnancies. There is no treatment, and the baby dies at birth or within a few days. The abnormality can be detected by **ultrasound** and **amniocentesis** tests in early pregnancy.

The cause of anencephaly is unknown, but there is a genetic link. The risk is reduced if a women who may become pregnant starts taking folic acid supplements from the time she stops using contraception until the end of the 12th week of pregnancy.

A much higher than usual dose of folic acid, taken under medical supervision, can reduce the risk of a baby with anencephaly in women who have a family history of the abnormality.
SEE ALSO *Pregnancy and problems*

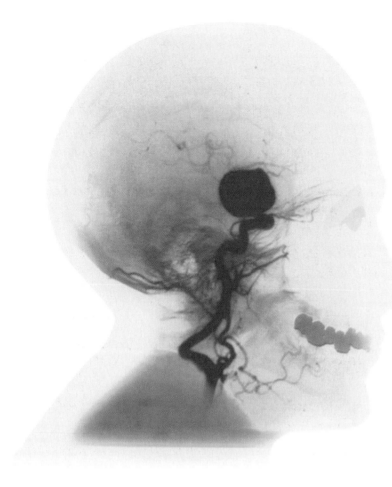

Aneurysm

An aneurysm is a swelling that develops in a diseased or weakened artery. It can form anywhere in the body, but most often occurs in the aorta (the main artery of the chest and abdomen). It is more common among people over the age of 55, especially men.

Sometimes aneurysms form in the blood vessels supplying the brain. Usually these are present from birth (congenital aneurysms), but they may form at sites of blood vessel weakness in older people, particularly those with high blood pressure.

Often there is no evidence of a cerebral aneurysm until it ruptures much later in life, causing a subarachnoid haemorrhage. This is a rare cause of sudden, unexpected death in young adults. Survivors may be left with varying degrees of neurological damage.

SYMPTOMS

Many aneurysms have no symptoms and are discovered only through routine examinations and X-rays. Aneurysms in the chest may put pressure on surrounding tissues and interfere with heart function, causing chest or back pain.

CAUSES

The most common cause of an aneurysm is **atheroma** (degenerative change) of the wall of the artery, but it is often associated with high blood pressure (hypertension). The cause of congenital aneurysm is unknown.

TREATMENT

If you suspect an aneurysm, seek medical advice urgently. A ruptured aortic aneurysm may cause kidney failure and stroke and can be fatal. Others may remain symptomless for many years, but when they develop, the risk of rupture has to be balanced against any risks of repair by surgery.

What a doctor may do

If there are symptoms, a doctor will investigate to see whether the aneurysm can be repaired by surgery. Doctors may choose not to treat symptomless aneurysms.

Aneurysms over 5cm (2in) wide can be repaired with synthetic tubing to prevent rupturing of the artery.

PREVENTION

The most effective prevention is to adopt a healthy lifestyle with regular exercise. Keep to a healthy weight, do not smoke, and restrict alcohol intake to 21–28 units a week for men and 14–21 units a week for women. Men over 60 with a family history of aortic aneurysm should request ultrasound screening. A national screening programme may be imminent.

Angina pectoris

Angina pectoris is chest pain caused by shortage of oxygen in the heart muscles. By far the most common cause is coronary artery disease that develops in middle age. The arteries that supply the heart become narrowed by deposits (plaques) containing cholesterol, so that blood flow is reduced. Other causative conditions include anaemia, thyroid disease and very fast or slow heart rates.

The condition is aggravated by exertion or stress because these increase demands on the heart. Other triggers include cold weather. It can be relieved by rest or medication.

SYMPTOMS

Angina is marked by a heavy, cramping pain, resembling the effect of a tight band, behind the breastbone. The pain may spread to the neck, jaw or left arm, and occasionally to the right arm. Other symptoms associated with angina include breathlessness, dizziness, sweating, nausea and vomiting.

TREATMENT

If you notice chest pain or severe breathlessness on exertion, consult a doctor. If the pain becomes more frequent, or recurs during minor exertion or when resting, seek medical help urgently. Unstable angina may lead to a heart attack. If an angina attack lasts for more than 15 minutes, it is important that an ambulance is called for.

What a doctor may do

Medication relieves symptoms and reduces the risk of heart attack. In severe cases, coronary artery intervention (**angioplasty** or **coronary bypass**) may be needed. But in the first instance your doctor may do the following.

■ Examine your heart and chest, and check your blood pressure, pulse, height and weight.

■ Order blood tests for anaemia, diabetes, kidney or liver abnormalities that might affect the severity of angina or the treatment that is chosen.

■ Arrange for a 'fasting' blood test. Restricting your consumption to water only for ten hours before the test enables a detailed analysis of cholesterol levels.

■ Arrange an electrocardiogram (**ECG** or heart tracing) to detect any heart damage that may have occurred.

■ Arrange an exercise tolerance (stress) test to show how the heart copes under stress. This is used to confirm the diagnosis.

■ Arrange an ultrasound scan.

■ Book a chest X-ray.

■ Arrange a coronary **angiography**.

■ Order a radio-isotope (thallium) scan of heart function if other tests do not prove conclusive.

PREVENTION

■ Lose weight (see **Body mass index**).

■ Stop smoking.

■ Drink within safe alcohol limits (14–21 units per week for women, 21–28 for men).

■ Walk briskly for 20 minutes five times a week (stop or slow down if doing this brings on any symptoms).

■ Adopt a healthier diet (see **Diet**).

■ Eat oily fish twice a week.

■ Lower stress levels.

■ Keep blood pressure down to 140/80.

■ In diabetics, good blood sugar control reduces the progression of coronary heart disease.

OUTLOOK

Adopting a healthier lifestyle and appropriate treatment will usually reduce angina symptoms and can also cut the risk of heart attacks, stroke and other circulatory diseases, which are more common in angina sufferers.

SEE ALSO *Arteries and disorders; Heart and circulatory system; Hypertension*

CONTACT **British Heart Foundation** 14 Fitzhardinge Street, London W1H 6DH 0845 708 070 (www.bhf.org.uk)

Drug treatments for angina

There are a variety of drugs prescribed for angina pectoris. These may vary according to the specific symptoms and the required action.

DRUG	BENEFITS	POSSIBLE SIDE EFFECTS
Glyceryl trinitrate (GTN) spray or tablets to use under the tongue	Dilates the coronary arteries and reduces heart and blood pressure	Headache or dizziness
GTN patches, isosorbide mono- or dinitrate tablets	Longer-acting form of nitrate; lowers blood pressure	Headaches, but they often reduce after the first few days
Beta-blockers, eg atenolol, metoprolol	Enable the heart to work more efficiently; reduce risk in raised blood pressure and after heart attacks	Cold extremities, fatigue; cannot be used in asthma. Sudden withdrawal may trigger severe angina
Calcium-channel blockers, eg amlodipine, diltiazem, verapamil	Improve heart muscle function; lower blood pressure	Headaches, ankle swelling. May aggravate heart failure
Potassium-channel activator, eg nicorandil	Dilates coronary arteries; lowers blood pressure	Headache, dizziness
Aspirin, clopidogrel or warfarin	Make blood less likely to clot	Internal bleeding
Statins or fibrates, eg atorvastatin	Lower cholesterol levels	Rarely, muscle or liver damage

Angiography

Angiography is an X-ray designed to ascertain the shape or direction of an artery. A dye is injected into the artery, and this shows up on the X-ray. It is used to diagnose problems in coronary artery disease and in peripheral artery disease (see **Arteries and disorders**).

The test is painless, once local anaesthetic has been injected to 'freeze' the skin around the artery in the groin or front of the elbow. A long, thin tube (catheter) is inserted into an artery and guided to the correct artery using an X-ray video camera. In coronary angiography, this will be the right or left coronary arteries.

Dye is flushed along the catheter into the artery, and X-ray 'snapshots' are taken immediately; these clearly show any areas of narrowing or blockage.

SEE ALSO *Heart and circulatory system*

Angio-oedema

Angio-oedema is a swelling of the skin and mucous membranes, caused by an excess of **histamine** released by the body in an allergic reaction. The eyes, face, lips and tongue may swell, restricting breathing. Bee and wasp stings may cause angio-oedema in people sensitive to them. Associated symptoms include headache, painful joints, the sensation of a lump in the throat, wheezing, shortness of breath, vomiting, diarrhoea and abdominal pain.

SEE ALSO *Allergies; Nettle rash*

Angioplasty

Angioplasty is a surgical technique used to widen blood vessels that have been narrowed or blocked as a result of arterial disease of the heart, the limbs or internal organs. In this condition, fatty deposits (atheroma), build up on the artery walls and restrict blood flow. Angioplasty is widely used for dilating the arteries supplying the heart – this is known as a coronary angioplasty.

WHAT'S INVOLVED
'Balloon' angioplasty, the most common technique used in the UK, generally requires overnight admission to hospital. Under local **anaesthetic**, a catheter (a narrow, flexible tube) with a tiny balloon attached to its end is inserted into the artery of the leg. It is guided under **X-ray** control to the narrowed coronary artery and then inflated. This procedure stretches the affected part of the artery, allowing the blood to flow through unrestricted. The balloon is then deflated and the catheter withdrawn.

Angioplasties are successful in most cases, and can be repeated if the artery becomes blocked or narrowed again. Sometimes a synthetic tube or coil known as a stent is inserted into the artery to keep it open; angioplasty can also be used after **coronary artery bypass grafts**.

OTHER TREATMENTS
Heavily diseased artery sections may not be suitable for balloon angioplasty. Alternative ways of clearing blocked arteries include using a rotoblator, a revolving burr that drills through the deposits. Sometimes a laser is used to break up the deposits.

SEE ALSO *Arteries and disorders*

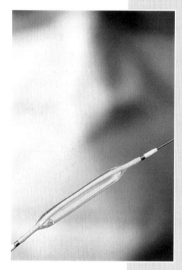

▲ **Balloon therapy**
A surgeon prepares to thread a catheter and balloon into an artery. The 'balloon' is then inflated to widen the narrowed artery.

Animals and health

While animals are often good for your health, they can also spread diseases. Rigorous hygiene and careful pet care reduce the risks.

Relationships with pets can benefit both adults and children, and pets are routinely welcomed into children's and old people's homes. But all animal lovers should be aware that people can catch diseases and parasitic infections from their pets and other animals.

ANIMAL BENEFITS
Research has shown that contact with pets has many positive effects.
- It decreases feelings of isolation and loneliness.
- It can lower blood pressure and blood cholesterol levels.
- It helps to develop patterns of nurturing behaviour in children.
- It can reduce agitation and depression in people with Alzheimer's disease.
- It helps older people to cope better with stress.
- It decreases the mortality rate after a heart attack by three per cent.
- Affection from animals can boost self-esteem.

ALLERGIES
Diseases transmitted from animals to people are known as zoonoses. Some can be extremely dangerous. One of the most common problems caused by pets is **hay fever,** or allergic rhinitis, which in turn may lead to **asthma.** In this case, the allergen is dander, tiny scales of dog and cat skin. Sometimes an allergy to dander or animal fur can also cause an allergic form of **eczema.**

INFECTIONS
Contact with animal faeces can lead to infective material being transferred to the mouth. The two main disorders transmitted in this way are both parasitic diseases: toxocariasis and toxoplasmosis.

Toxocariasis is caused by a small worm that lives in the intestines of cats and dogs. In people, the worms migrate to many of the body's organs and can cause blindness.

Toxoplasmosis is much more common and less dangerous that toxocariasis, except in pregnancy. The parasite responsible, *Toxoplasma gondii,* lives in the intestines of cats. Some people

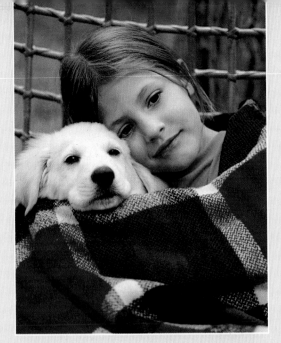

experience mild symptoms, such as a raised temperature, tiredness and swollen lymph nodes in the neck and armpits; occasionally, there may be retinitis and other eye problems.

Mild toxoplasmosis does not generally require treatment, though antimalarial drugs may be given when there is retinitis. However, people with disorders of the immune system, and infants who have received the infection from their mothers during pregnancy are at more serious risk. Possible complications include **encephalitis**, **myocarditis** and damage to the eyes and brain. A toxoplasmosis infection that occurs early in pregnancy can cause a miscarriage or stillbirth; if the infection occurs later on, it can cause mental or physical damage to the baby. For

this reason, pregnant women are urged to observe scrupulous hygiene, and some authorities advise them to avoid cats.

BITES AND SCRATCHES

Domestic animals normally play host to a large number of bacteria, especially in the mouth and on the paws, and from time to time to fleas, ticks and mites. For this reason, any bite or scratch from a dog or cat should be medically examined in case **antibiotics** or an antitetanus injection are needed (see also **Tetanus**). Consult a doctor if you are bitten while abroad, or if the dog that bit you seemed crazed or ill. **Rabies** is still prevalent in Europe.

A scratch from a cat infected by the bacterium *Bartonella henselae*, spread from cat to cat by fleas, can cause a condition called **cat-scratch fever**. It usually affects only people aged under 21 years, primarily children. The symptoms develop after an incubation period of between one and two weeks. A pustule develops at the site of the scratch; then, a few days later, lymph nodes near the scratch become swollen, and there is often fever, tiredness and loss of appetite. Sometimes antibiotics are given, but generally cat-scratch fever clears up on its own in a few months. The infection cannot be passed from one person to another. The best form of prevention is to de-flea cats regularly.

OTHER RISKS

Contact with dogs and cats can also cause a number of fungal infections. The most common of these is the **fungal infection** tinea. Bites from insects living in animal fur can transmit a number of diseases, all known as **typhus**.

There are also risks to people who come into contact with agricultual and other animals. **Leptospirosis**, also known as Weil's disease, can be caught from bacteria expelled in the urine of rats; while **psittacosis**, a flu-like disorder, can be contracted from poultry, pigeons and parrots. **Brucellosis**, a bacterial condition, is now rare, but remains a hazard for those who work with cattle, pigs and goats.

SEE ALSO *Parasites and parasitic diseases*

CONTACT **Pets As Therapy** 3 Grange Farm Cottages, Wycombe Road, Saunderton, Princes Risborough, Bucks HP27 9NS 0870 240 1239 (www.petsastherapy.org) The organization arranges therapeutic visits to hospitals, hospices and nursing homes by volunteers with their dogs and cats.

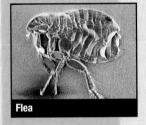
Flea

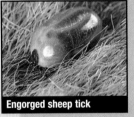
Engorged sheep tick

Animal care checklist

Stick to these guidelines so that you and your pets stay healthy.

Do

✓ Worm your pets regularly, especially if you have children or are pregnant.

✓ Dispose of animal faeces immediately.

✓ Keep pet food, utensils and bowls separate from your food and kitchen equipment.

✓ Wash and clean any scratch from a pet and treat with antiseptic cream.

Don't

✗ Forget to take your pets for regular checkups with the vet.

✗ Neglect to use veterinary flea and tick preventives regularly.

✗ Allow pets to lick your or your children's faces.

Ankle and problems

The ankle is a joint between the uppermost bone in the foot (the talus) and the two bones of the lower leg (the tibia and the fibula), which are bound together by strong ligaments. As it is a hinge joint, the ankle allows movement only in one plane – up and down. Other movements (such as rotation of the ankle) involve bones in the foot itself.

SPRAINED ANKLE

The commonest injury is a sprain of the ligament at its outside edge (the lateral ligament), which results from twisting the ankle. This causes pain, swelling and bruising, which can be severe.

Treat a sprained ankle with rest, by applying an ice pack and compression bandaging, and by elevating it. For more severe sprains, seek medical opinion to rule out a fracture or a torn ligament. A severely sprained ankle may have to be strapped up for two or three weeks.

BROKEN ANKLE

Excessive, violent twisting of the ankle can cause a fracture. Most ankle fractures involve the lower end of the tibia and/or fibula.

If you fall onto your feet from a great height, you may cause a vertical compression injury of the ankle. A combined fracture and dislocation of the ankle is known as a 'Pott's fracture'; this occurs when the lower fibula (and sometimes the tibia as well) fractures and the ligaments tear so that the ankle joint dislocates.

Simple fractures are treated by immobilizing the joint in plaster. Severe injuries may require a screw to be surgically inserted into the joint.

SEE ALSO *Achilles tendon rupture; Arthritis; Bruises; Club foot and hand; Sports injuries and therapy*

Ankylosing spondylitis

Ankylosing spondylitis is a disease of the joints, mainly affecting the spine. The joints become stiff and inflamed and, if left untreated, may fuse together and become rigid. In the UK about one in 200 people have the condition, which is most likely to develop in adults when they are in their early 20s. Those affected are usually men. Spinal joints are the main ones involved, but in some cases the shoulders, hips and knees may be affected. There is no definite known cause, although there is a genetic link (see **Genetics and genetic disorders**).

SYMPTOMS

Ankylosing spondylitis progresses slowly over many years. Symptoms include:
- repeated attacks of lower back pain in a healthy, fit person aged between 20 and 40;
- early-morning back pain and stiffness, which can move down one or both legs;
- increasing stiffness of the whole spine;
- tenderness over the hip joints;
- limited chest expansion.

TREATMENT

If you suffer from several symptoms, seek medical advice. Also, if there is a family history of the disease, it is advisable to consult your doctor about tests – they can assist in early diagnosis, allowing prompt treatment.

What a doctor may do
- X-ray the lower part of your back and carry out a blood test. If the diagnosis is confirmed, your doctor may refer you to hospital.
- Prescribe painkillers and anti-inflammatory drugs to relieve the symptoms and slow down the progress of the disease.
- Arrange **physiotherapy**, which can help to strengthen spinal muscles, mobilize the joints and stretch ligaments.
- Suggest a hip replacement (see **Joint replacement**) if hip joints are badly affected.
- Arrange **radiotherapy** occasionally, if pain is severe and uncontrollable.

What you can do
- A daily exercise programme helps to relieve pain and maintain mobility. Swimming is an excellent form of exercise to help to keep the body as supple as possible.
- Lie face down for 20 minutes at the beginning and end of the day.
- Sleep on a firm mattress.
- Keep to a healthy weight.
- Try to maintain good posture (see **Back and back pain**).

Complementary therapies
Hydrotherapy, shiatsu, t'ai chi ch'uan and meditation may all be beneficial. **Acupuncture** may relieve pain.

COMPLICATIONS

Long-term ankylosing spondylitis may cause the spine to become rigid, leading to curvature (kyphosis) which, with neck distortion, can be extremely disabling.

Other potential complications of the disease include ulcerative colitis, Crohn's disease and certain heart defects. Iritis (inflammation of the iris) occurs in 40 per cent of cases.

OUTLOOK

For cases that are treated early with anti-inflammatory drugs and physiotherapy, the outlook is usually good.

Ankylosing spondylitis may interfere with work or physical activity.

CONTACT **National Ankylosing Spondylitis Society** PO Box 179, Mayfield, East Sussex TN20 6ZL (01435) 873527 (www.nass.co.uk)

Anorexia nervosa

People with anorexia nervosa have an intense fear of putting on weight. The condition can develop when a person focuses on controlling food intake and body shape as a way of coping with painful feelings.

The clearest sign of anorexia is severe weight loss. Sufferers weigh at least 15 per cent less than is usual for their age and height. The condition is more obvious but rarer than **bulimia nervosa**. People can fluctuate between the two conditions. Most sufferers are girls and young women, although men can be affected and even children as young as seven or eight.

People with anorexia restrict the amount they eat and drink not because they are not hungry, but because they cannot allow themselves to satisfy their appetites. They have mixed feelings about 'giving up' their illness because their eating habits have become a way of coping with their emotional problems.

The causes are varied. Some people are more vulnerable due to their genetic make-up or personalities. People with low self-esteem, anxiety or depression may focus on avoiding food to cope with stress or pressure. Traumatic events such as the death of a friend or relative, sexual abuse or divorce can trigger the illness.

HOW OTHERS CAN HELP

The first step is to see a doctor, but it can be hard for people with anorexia to accept that they need help – and they must want to get better before any good can result. Friends and family should try to build a relationship of trust with sufferers without forcing them to get help. The focus should be on emotions rather than on food or weight. It may be useful to suggest that individuals get help to deal with the feelings at the root of the anorexia, rather than the anorexia itself.

A GP can refer someone with anorexia to a specialist in **eating disorders**. **Counselling, psychotherapy** or family therapy may address underlying emotional problems, or a psychologist may provide **cognitive behaviour therapy**. When a person is dangerously underweight, the doctor may advise a spell in a hospital or clinic. Music, dance, drama or **art therapy** may benefit those who find it hard to express themselves in words. **Aromatherapy, massage** and **reflexology** can help people to feel more connected with their body.

The Eating Disorders Association provides help and support for people with anorexia, and their family and friends.

LONG-TERM EFFECTS AND RECOVERY

Refusing food over a long period can lead to malnutrition and, sometimes, death. Women can find it difficult to become pregnant and may develop **osteoporosis** (brittle bones). But many of the physical problems associated with anorexia can be reversed once the body is given proper nourishment. Long-term psychological solutions depend on sufferers coming to understand the origins of their eating distress – and finding other ways of coping with their feelings and with stressful situations.

> CONTACT **Eating Disorders Association**
> First Floor, Wensum House, 103 Prince of Wales Road, Norwich NR1 1DW; helpline 0845 634 1414; youthline (0845) 634 7650 (www.edauk.com)
> **Mind** 15–19 Broadway, London E15 4BQ
> Mind*info*line 0845 766 0163 9.15am–5.15pm Mon–Fri (www.mind.org.uk)

Anorexia affects one in 100 girls and young women in the UK.

▼ **Keeping warm**
As the body of an anorexic struggles to adapt to decreasing amounts of fat and muscle, it develops a fine covering of hair to help retain body heat.

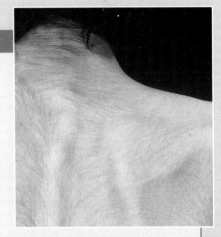

Factfile

Signs of anorexia

Many emotional and behavioural changes are linked with anorexia, including:

■ an intense fear of gaining weight;

■ a belief by sufferers that they are fat when they are underweight;

■ mood swings;

■ secrecy in regard to food;

■ rituals such as cutting food into tiny pieces;

■ wearing big, baggy clothes;

■ exercising obsessively;

■ vomiting or taking laxatives.

Girls and women with anorexia often have irregular then absent periods, while men are likely to suffer a loss of libido. Other physical signs are:

■ constipation and abdominal pains;

■ downy hair on the body;

■ feeling cold, due to poor circulation;

■ dry, rough, discoloured skin;

■ swollen stomach, face and ankles;

■ dizzy spells and fainting;

■ restlessness and hyperactivity.

Anoxia

Anoxia refers to a complete break in oxygen supply to the tissues of an organ even where there is an adequate supply of blood; the term 'hypoxia' means a reduction in oxygen supply to an organ. Despite the difference in meaning, the two words are often used interchangeably to describe a decline in oxygen supply. Some 20 per cent of the body's supply of oxygen is used by the brain. As a result, it is particularly sensitive to anoxia or hypoxia, which can lead to coma or seizures and, if left untreated, death.

CAUSES

The conditions and events that may adversely affect the supply of oxygen to an organ include:
- a heart attack;
- a severe asthma attack;
- an adverse reaction to an anaesthetic;
- inhalation of smoke or carbon monoxide;
- exposure to high altitude;
- strangulation or suffocation;
- poisoning.

TREATMENT

Treatment may include artificial ventilation, oxygen therapy and investigation of any underlying causes.

SEE ALSO *Artificial respiration; Oxygen*

Antacids

Antacids are drugs that neutralize excess acid in the stomach and in so doing raise its pH level. They relieve the symptoms of **indigestion**, gastritis and heartburn (caused by regurgitation of acid and enzymes).

Commonly used antacids include salts of aluminium (sucralfate and aluminium hydroxide), salts of magnesium (for example, magnesium carbonate) and other basic salts (for example, sodium bicarbonate).

ADVICE ON USAGE

- Antacids containing high levels of sodium should not be taken by anyone on a sodium-restricted diet.
- Antacids can interfere with the absorption of other drugs.
- Antacids should not be used regularly to relieve abdominal pain, except on medical advice, because they may mask the symptoms of stomach cancer.
- Bicarbonates and carbonates can cause flatulence and belching. Some aluminium-containing antacids can cause constipation, while magnesium-containing antacids can cause diarrhoea – so the two types are often taken together.

SEE ALSO *Diet; Drugs, medicinal*

Antepartum haemorrhage

Antepartum haemorrhage means bleeding from the womb in pregnancy. It may signal a serious problem, so the pregnant woman should seek medical advice promptly if bleeding occurs. Slight spotting around the time of the first missed period is common, but more pronounced bleeding may indicate a complication involving the placenta or a threatened **miscarriage**.

SEE ALSO *Placenta praevia; Pregnancy and problems*

Anthrax

Anthrax is a disease of farm animals that occasionally spreads to human beings. It may be fatal if left untreated, but is very rare in the UK.

The anthrax bacterium attacks either the skin (cutaneous anthrax) or the lungs (pulmonary anthrax). People may become infected through cuts or sores if handling products from infected animals, or by inhaling large quantities of infected spores. Cutaneous anthrax causes swelling and deep ulcers, but is easily treated in its earliest stages with penicillin. Pulmonary anthrax causes severe breathing problems and pneumonia, and is fatal in most cases.

Antibacterials

Antibacterials are **drugs** used to treat infections caused by bacteria. Most antibacterials work by preventing bacteria from growing and multiplying. The vast majority are available only on prescription. They include **antibiotics** and synthetic drugs, including:
- sulphonamides, such as trimethoprim – used to treat, for example, infections of the urinary tract and chronic bronchitis;
- sulphones, such as dapsone – used in leprosy treatment;
- quinolones, such as ciprofloxacin – used to treat infections of the urinary, gastro-intestinal and respiratory tracts, especially in people who are allergic to penicillin or whose infection is resistant to standard antibiotics.

ADVICE ON USAGE

Most antibacterial medication is taken by mouth, in liquid or tablet form. It may also be given by injection and carried by the blood to the site of infection. Others can be applied externally to treat infections of superficial tissues (close to the skin surface) such as the skin or the eye.

Antibacterials usually take several days to eliminate bacteria from the body, and the full course of treatment should be completed even if you feel better before you have finished it. This is because if any bacteria remain they may multiply rapidly and develop resistance to the drug so causing a re-infection.

Some people may be allergic to certain antibacterials – in particular, penicillin.

SEE ALSO **Bacterial infections**

Antibiotics

Antibiotics, naturally secreted by micro-organisms such as fungi, yeasts and moulds, inhibit the growth of other micro-organisms. But the term 'antibiotics' is often used synonymously with **antibacterials** to describe **drugs** used to treat infections.

The first medicinal antibiotic, **penicillin**, was introduced in 1941. Since then, antibiotics have become some of the most widely prescribed types of drug in modern medicine.

Certain antibiotics, such as tetracyclines and cephalosporins, are known as broad-spectrum antibiotics and can be used against a wide variety of bacteria. Narrow-spectrum antibiotics treat infections caused by a few bacteria types. A broad-spectrum antibiotic may be prescribed until laboratory tests have identified the bacterium responsible for an infection, whereupon a more specific, narrow-spectrum antibiotic may be substituted.

Some antibiotics, for example, nystatin, are effective against fungi and yeasts that cause disease (see **Antifungals**). Because some are toxic to certain cancer cells they can be used in **chemotherapy**, and some are used as immuno-suppressant drugs. No antibiotics are effective against viruses.

RISKS OF OVERUSE

The extensive use of antibiotics has resulted in antibiotic resistance – that is, certain bacteria have become resistant to the effects of particular antibiotics. An antibiotic-resistant 'super-infection' called methicillin-resistant *Staphylococcus aureus* (MRSA) is now a major problem in hospitals (see **Iatrogenic disease**). Another risk of antibiotic treatment is the disturbance of the normal micro-organisms in the body, which can lead to gastro-intestinal upsets and **thrush**. Antibiotics can reduce the effectiveness of the contraceptive pill.

In the picture below, antibodies surround a foreign cell before destroying it; in the picture beneath this, autoantibodies are seen clustering in the blood of a person with the autoimmune disease systemic lupus erythematosus (SLE).

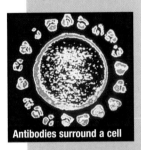

Antibodies surround a cell

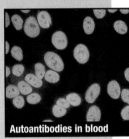

Autoantibodies in blood

Antibodies

Molecules made by the immune system as a defence against foreign proteins are called antibodies. In a healthy person, antibodies recognize foreign cells, such as invading micro-organisms, and initiate their destruction.

In **autoimmune diseases**, autoantibodies are produced and these can attack and damage the body's own tissues.

SEE ALSO **Healing; Immune system and disorders**

Anticoagulants

Anticoagulants are substances that prevent the clotting (coagulation) of blood and inhibit the formation of blood clots. They are used medicinally to 'thin the blood' – that is, to maintain normal blood flow and to prevent and treat blood clots in conditions such as embolism and thrombosis, especially after surgery.

The body's own natural anticoagulant is heparin, which can also be injected as a drug. There are also synthetic anticoagulants taken by mouth, such as warfarin sodium, which inhibits the action of the blood-clotting vitamin K.

People who take anticoagulants are monitored mainly to ensure that the dose is at the right level to achieve sufficient anticoagulation without a high risk of bleeding. Profuse bleeding following injury is a common hazard when taking anticoagulant medication.

SEE ALSO **Blood and disorders; Drugs, medicinal**

Anticonvulsants

The commonest use of anticonvulsant **drugs** is to prevent or reduce the severity of seizures in **epilepsy**. They are also used to prevent or control **convulsions**, for example, after drug or chemical poisoning.

Benzodiazepines such as diazepam work for most convulsive states. However, epilepsy requires specialist drugs, such as valproic acid derivatives, phenytoin and phenobarbital.

Many anticonvulsants can cause fetal abnormalities if taken during pregnancy.

Antidepressants

Antidepressants are drugs used to relieve the symptoms of clinical **depression**. There are several different groups of antidepressants, but they all work by changing levels of chemicals in the brain, particularly serotonin and noradrenaline, in areas that regulate mood.

The two oldest groups are tricyclics (eg amitriptyline) and MAOIs (monoamine-oxidase inhibitors, eg phenelzine and isocarboxazid). The most recent antidepressants are the SSRIs (selective serotonin re-uptake inhibitors, such as Prozac (fluoxetine). SSRIs are prescribed more frequently because they have fewer side effects and interactions than older antidepressants.

Antidepressants must usually be taken for up to two weeks before they start to work, and for up to six to eight weeks before their full effect is experienced. Treatment must be stopped gradually, otherwise withdrawal symptoms may occur. If changing from one type of antidepressant to another, there must be a 'washout period' of several weeks.

Antidepressants can cause serious reactions if taken with a number of other drugs and herbal remedies (eg St John's Wort).
SEE ALSO *Depression; Drugs, medicinal*

In the UK, as many as 20 per cent of people may suffer from some form of depression during their lives.

Antidotes

Antidotes are medicines used to counteract toxic effects – for example, acetylcysteine is taken for paracetamol overdose, naloxone for heroin overdose and **antivenoms** for snake or insect bites. Some antidotes hasten the removal of a drug or poison from the body; for example, heavy metal poisoning is treated with chelating agents (chemical compounds that bind metal ions and so relieve symptoms).
SEE ALSO *Drugs, medicinal*

Antifungals

Antifungals are drugs used to treat fungal infections – that is, infections caused by a variety of yeasts, moulds and mushrooms. To treat superficial, contained infections such as athlete's foot, antifungals are applied to the affected area as a cream or solution. For severe infections affecting the entire body they are given by mouth or injection.

Examples of antifungal drugs are azoles (eg clotrimazole, metronidazole), tolnaftate, nystatin, amphotericin B and griseofulvin.
SEE ALSO *Drugs, medicinal; Fungal infections*

Antigens

Antigens are any substances that, when introduced into the body, are recognized as foreign and stimulate the production of an immune response. **Antibodies** and specialized cells, such as lymphocytes, are then marshalled in defence. Common antigens include the proteins carried on the surface of pollen grains, bacteria and viruses.
SEE ALSO *Allergies; Immune system and disorders*

Antihistamines

Antihistamines are drugs used to treat allergic reactions, particularly allergic rhinitis (eg **hay fever**), allergic **conjunctivitis** and allergic skin reactions such as a **rash**. Antihistamines block sites in the body at which the natural substance histamine causes allergic symptoms. Some antihistamines also prevent nausea and are used for motion sickness, vertigo or to prevent vomiting caused by chemotherapy. Some are sedating and are used in preparations for coughs and colds and to aid sleep.

Side effects of some antihistamines include dry mouth, blurred vision and possibly drowsiness, so avoid driving or operating dangerous machinery if you are taking them. Newer antihistamines, such as cetirizine, are less likely to make you drowsy.
SEE ALSO *Drugs, medicinal*

Antioxidants

Antioxidants are substances that slow down or prevent deterioration, damage or destruction in the body caused by oxidation – a process that produces rogue molecules called free radicals.

The body has an army of antioxidant molecules in the form of enzymes. When these antioxidants can no longer control the numbers of free radicals produced by oxidation, the body may be prone to diseases and conditions including age spots (see **Skin and disorders**), **arthritis** and skin **cancer** as well as heart and liver disease, so it pays to eat foods that replenish the body's supply of antioxidants.

Many everyday foods – particularly fruit, vegetables, seeds, nuts and whole grains – contain a range of antioxidant nutrients with the power to augment the body's natural antioxidant capacity. Such nutrients include:
■ vitamin A, found in orange and dark green fruit and vegetables;
■ vitamin C, found in many different types of fruit and vegetables;

- vitamin E, found in plant oils, cereals, nuts and seeds;
- zinc, found in seafood, fish and seeds.
  Antioxidant nutrients can also be taken in **vitamin dietary supplements**.

SEE ALSO *Diet*

Antiperspirants

Antiperspirants are used medically to reduce excessive sweating (hyperhidrosis), for instance, when some disorder of the sweat glands causes constant and streaming perspiration. Fresh perspiration is odourless but it creates an environment in which bacteria and fungi can thrive. This produces chemical changes that result in unpleasant odours.

SEE ALSO *Body odour*

Antiseptics

Antiseptics are substances that inhibit the growth or reproduction of micro-organisms. They can be used to prevent infection, decomposition and similar damaging changes in living tissue. In medicine, they are used as mouthwashes, skin solutions and wipes to limit the spread of disease.

SEE ALSO *Drugs, medicinal*

Antiserum

Antiserum (also called immune serum) is a preparation of blood fluid that contains particular **antibodies**. These antibodies, once injected, provide immunity to a specific disease. This is known as passive immunity, and is a different process to that used by vaccines, which provoke the body to produce its own antibodies to give immunity (see **Immunization**). Antiserums contain proteins that are foreign to the body, so an allergic reaction can occur.

SEE ALSO *Drugs, medicinal*

Antitoxin

Antitoxin is a type of **antiserum**. It is usually obtained from horses that have been immunized against a particular toxin-producing organism. Antitoxin is used to treat people who have been affected by a poison of biological origin. There are, for example, antitoxins to treat diphtheria, botulism and snake or spider venom.

SEE ALSO *Antivenom; Drugs, medicinal*

Antivenom

Antivenom (also known as antivenin) is a type of **antitoxin** that works as an **antidote** to the poison from a snakebite, or to the bite or sting of another poisonous animal. Usually, it is a preparation of venom-neutralizing antibodies in **antiserum** and is given intravenously as emergency first aid.

SEE ALSO *Drugs, medicinal*

Anus and problems

The anus is the opening at the lower end of the digestive tract, through which stools (faeces) pass during defecation. It is connected to the rectum by the anal canal, which is about 4cm (1⅜in) long.

Normally, the anus is held closed by two bands of muscle that run around it: the external and internal sphincters. The external sphincter is under voluntary control – it can be relaxed deliberately. The internal one can only be relaxed by the autonomic nervous system, which operates without conscious control.

The lower half of the anal canal has the same number of sensory nerve endings as normal skin; the upper half has no sensory nerve endings and, like the intestines, only responds to increases in tension from the pressure of faeces. For this reason cancer of the lower bowel does not cause pain until it has spread to the lower anal canal.

WHAT CAN GO WRONG?
- The most common problem to affect the anus is **haemorrhoids** – painful swollen veins that may develop either inside or outside the anus.
- Anal fissures are small tears in the lining of the anus, usually caused when a person suffering from **constipation** passes hard stools. Anal fissures are treated with antibiotics and medicated creams.
- Bacteria can invade the tissues of the anal canal to form an anal **abscess**, especially when there is also **Crohn's disease** or a disorder that reduces the efficiency of the immune system. Doctors will drain the abscess.
- Crohn's disease or the presence of an abscess make it likely that an anal fistula will develop. This is a small channel that opens between the rectum and the skin near the anus and is treated with antibiotics and surgery.
- Itching in the anus (*pruritus ani*) can occur for no apparent reason or can be a sign of an infestation by **threadworms**.
- Very rarely, children are born without an anal opening. The condition, called an imperforate anus, affects one in 5000 births and is corrected by surgery.

Anxiety

Anxiety is a normal reaction to **stress**. After a stressful event, the anxiety will usually go away. But anxiety becomes a problem when it persists beyond an event or interferes with your day-to-day life and your relationships.

Anxiety can feed on itself, so that the sufferer worries about feeling anxious which then increases the anxiety. It can lead to **insomnia** or **panic attacks** or may develop into **depression,** an **obsession** or **phobia.**

SYMPTOMS

The symptoms of anxiety can take many forms:
- fearfulness and a pessimistic outlook;
- over-alertness or irritability;
- inability to relax or concentrate;
- tense muscles;
- headaches;
- raised heartbeat, high blood pressure and sweating;
- nausea, sickness or diarrhoea;
- insomnia.

CAUSES

The most common causes of persistent anxiety are stressful life events now or in the past, especially those connected with work, money, relationships, death or divorce.

Another important factor is family history: the way in which your parents cope with pressure and stress can influence the likelihood of your developing an anxiety problem.

Other causes include a poor diet, especially one that includes excess sugar or caffeine, **drug misuse** or the side effects of prescribed drugs.

TREATMENT

Consult a doctor if you are concerned that your anxiety is becoming overwhelming.

What a doctor may do
- Check for any underlying illness.
- Refer you to a counsellor or a psychologist for **cognitive behaviour therapy.** (See also **Psychological therapies.**)
- Prescribe **tranquillizers** or sleeping pills.

What you can do
Reassess your job, ambitions and lifestyle and make changes accordingly. It helps to identify the source of your anxiety – for example, bullying at work.

Complementary and other therapies
- **regular exercise, massage, aromatherapy, reflexology** or **hypnotherapy** may help you to relax and sleep better.
- Learn **relaxation** and breathing techniques from self-help tapes.
- Join a **yoga** or **meditation** class.

CONTACT **SANE**; helpline 0845 767 8000 (www.sane.org.uk)

Aorta and disorders

The aorta is the main artery in the body. It has a thick muscular wall and carries oxygenated blood from the heart to the peripheral arteries to supply the head, trunk, limbs and vital organs.

When oxygenated blood returns from the lungs, it is pumped through the left ventricle and aortic valve into the ascending aorta, where the coronary arteries branch off to supply the heart itself. The aortic valve stops blood from flowing back into the heart when it relaxes.

WHAT CAN GO WRONG

There are a number of conditions and disorders that can develop.

Abnormal development
The aortic valve and the aorta may develop abnormally in the fetus. This can happen in isolation or as part of a syndrome such as **Fallot's tetralogy.** If the aortic valve has two flaps instead of the normal three, it may thicken and stiffen, or it may leak in later life. This makes it harder for the left ventricle to pump blood into the aorta, and can lead to heart failure. In many cases, surgery can correct the condition.

Aortic regurgitation
The aortic valve may leak as a result of damage caused by rheumatic heart disease (see **Rheumatic fever**), heart attack (see **Myocardial infarction**) and several other conditions such as **rheumatoid arthritis.** There can also be a congenital weakness of the valve. Blood ebbs back into the left ventricle from the aorta after each heartbeat, increasing the heart's workload. This can lead to breathlessness or heart failure; drugs or artificial valve replacement may be needed.

Aortic stenosis
Narrowing of the aortic valve may be caused by rheumatic heart disease, or by hardening caused by calcium deposition, which occurs with ageing. This can cause fainting and breathlessness, and lead to **angina.** An artificial valve replacement is often needed to treat these symptoms, and strenuous activity may be harmful.

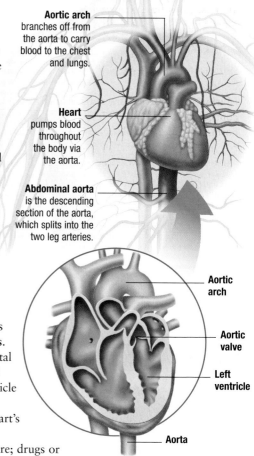

Aorta
The largest artery in the body, the aorta carries blood from the heart to other parts of the body.

Aortic arch branches off from the aorta to carry blood to the chest and lungs.

Heart pumps blood throughout the body via the aorta.

Abdominal aorta is the descending section of the aorta, which splits into the two leg arteries.

Aortic arch

Aortic valve

Left ventricle

Aorta

Coarctation of the aorta

Usually detected in childhood, coarctation of the aorta is a condition in which the aortic arch is abnormally narrowed. It affects one person in 1700, and unless the condition is corrected by surgery, 50 per cent of sufferers will die before the age of 30.

If coarctation is undetected until adulthood, raised blood pressure or premature heart failure may be the first clues to the condition.

Coarctation must be repaired; the narrowed section is cut out or replaced with an artificial graft, or widened by balloon **angioplasty**. One in ten cases recurs after surgery.

Aortic aneurysm

An aortic aneurysm is a localized swelling caused by weakness in the wall of the abdominal or thoracic aorta. Aneurysms of the abdominal aorta are commonly caused by **atheroma**, a degeneration of the walls of the arteries. Those in the thoracic aorta are more often caused by diseases that affect the wall of the aorta, such as Marfan's syndrome (see below). In both cases, the aneurysm may rupture, leading to internal bleeding.

Marfan's syndrome

Marfan's syndrome is a genetic disorder of connective tissue that produces weakness of the aorta. This leads to dilation of the aorta and results in stretching and leaking of the aortic valve. The wall of the aorta may tear, leading to death in early adulthood, unless the condition is detected by an **ultrasound** picture of the heart and aorta.

SEE ALSO *Heart and circulatory system*

CONTACT **Grown Up Congenital Heart Patients' Association**; helpline 0800 854759 (www.guch.demon.co.uk)
Marfan Association UK (01252) 810472 (www.marfan.org.uk)

Apathy

Apathy is a state of listlessness or fatigue in which the person affected seems to have lost interest in life. Simple tasks and decisions become very hard or impossible; the person may withdraw from any social contact or be unable to work.

Apathy may be short-lived and disappear by itself. Alternatively, it may be a symptom of an underlying problem such as **depression, Alzheimer's disease** or **schizophrenia**. It is sometimes the side effect of prescribed drugs or the result of a head injury or **stroke**. Treatment of the underlying condition should mean that the apathy dissipates.

Apgar score

The Apgar test was devised by the American paediatrician Dr Virginia Apgar to assess the physical condition of a newborn baby. One minute after the birth, and again at five minutes, the heartbeat, breathing, muscle tone, reflexes and skin colour are each given a score of zero, one or two. Most babies score between seven and ten; ten is ideal, but a score below seven indicates that the baby may need resuscitation.

SEE ALSO *Birth and problems*

Aphasia

The term 'aphasia' covers a wide range of language impairments caused by damage to the language-processing regions of the brain, usually due to head injury or **stroke**. In 95 per cent of people, the language areas lie in the left cerebral hemisphere. In the other five per cent, language is processed in either the right or both left and right sides. The form of aphasia depends on which part of the language area is affected. There are three common types.

Broca's aphasia involves an inability to express language and articulate sentences correctly. Speech tends to be minimal or disjointed, but comprehension is not greatly affected.

Wernicke's aphasia involves a difficulty in understanding language, despite the retention of normal intelligence in other ways. Speech is fluent, but the content is garbled or nonsensical.

Anomic aphasia involves a difficulty in retrieving words and using them with good comprehension and grammar.

SEE ALSO *Brain and nervous system; Cerebral haemorrhage; Head and injuries; Stroke*

Apnoea

Apnoea is a pause in breathing during sleep. It lasts between 10 and 30 seconds, and can cause problems both in babies and in adults. There is a possible link between apnoea in babies and cot death (**sudden infant death syndrome**).

In the UK, it affects one to two per cent of men and two per cent of women in middle age. The airways close during sleep and cause heavy snoring. To clear the blockage, the person wakes up (too briefly to remember doing so) 400–500 times a night. Apnoea can cause tiredness and mental health problems. It is associated with increased risk of heart disease and cardiac arrhythmias. Apnoea can be treated with a breathing aid worn at night.

SEE ALSO *Sleep disorders*

Apoplexy

Apoplexy is an old-fashioned term for severe **stroke** – a sudden loss of consciousness due to interruption of blood flow through the brain.

Appendix and appendicitis

The appendix is a tubular pouch in the large intestine about 9cm (3½in) in length. It has no known function. Appendicitis (inflammation of the appendix) can develop at any time, but is most prevalent in people aged between 8 and 25 years old. It is treated by surgical removal of the appendix, which very rarely has any damaging effect.

Acute appendicitis, which strikes its victims suddenly, is the most common reason for emergency surgery in developing countries.

Chronic (persistent or recurring) appendicitis is far less severe than the acute version of the condition, and may continue for several months before an operation becomes necessary.

SYMPTOMS

There is wide variation in the symptoms of appendicitis, and the condition can easily be confused with many other ailments.

In chronic appendicitis, symptoms may never develop beyond an indeterminate discomfort on the right-hand side of the abdomen. But in about half of all cases of acute appendicitis, the symptoms follow an established pattern.
- Initially, there is a feeling of discomfort around the navel.
- Within a few hours, a sharper, more constant pain develops around McBurney's point, which is two-thirds of the way along a line drawn between the navel and the right hip bone. The pain is worse on moving or coughing, and when pressure is released after McBurney's point is pressed.
- There may be a raised temperature, sickness and vomiting, sometimes accompanied by constipation or diarrhoea.
- If the appendix is pressing on the ureter, the urine may be bloodstained.

CAUSES

Sometimes the open end of the appendix gets blocked, causing swelling and infection. But the cause of appendicitis is often unknown.

TREATMENT

If you think that you may be suffering from the symptoms of appendicitis, there are several things you can do before seeking medical help.
- Lie still, holding a hot-water bottle over the painful area to ease discomfort.
- Do not eat or drink anything.
- Do not take painkillers, laxatives or other medication.

When to consult a doctor

If pain has persisted for more than three to four hours, call a doctor. Summon help earlier if the pain grows worse, becomes continuous or keeps you awake during the night.

What a doctor may do

If acute appendicitis is suspected, the doctor will probably send you to hospital immediately for observation or surgery. In some circumstances the doctor may decide to monitor your condition at home.

In cases of acute appendicitis, emergency surgery often proves necessary. Patients are usually discharged from hospital within two to three days after the operation if no subsequent complications occur.

If your condition is chronic rather than acute, surgery may not be necessary for several months.

PREVENTION

Eating a diet high in fibre may help to prevent appendicitis. The condition is less common in countries where a high-fibre diet is the norm.

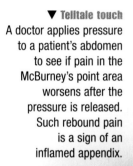

▼ **Telltale touch**
A doctor applies pressure to a patient's abdomen to see if pain in the McBurney's point area worsens after the pressure is released. Such rebound pain is a sign of an inflamed appendix.

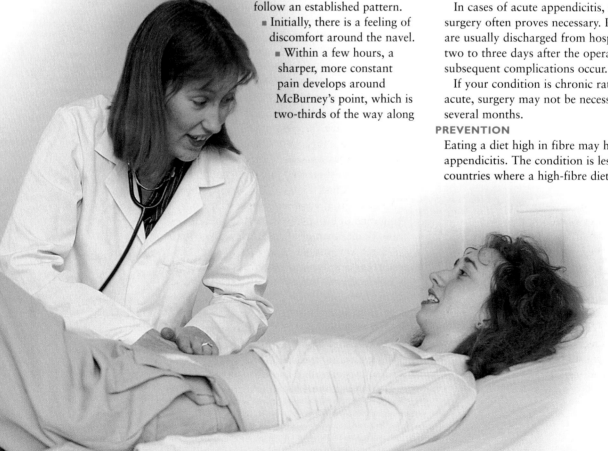

COMPLICATIONS

■ If treatment is delayed, there is a danger that the inflamed appendix may rupture, spilling its contents into the abdomen and causing the more serious condition of **peritonitis**. This occurs in about 20 per cent of cases.

■ A rupture may form an **abscess**, causing fever and increasing pain in the abdomen.

■ A ruptured appendix can also infect the blood, causing blood poisoning (**septicaemia**).

■ In women, the ovaries and Fallopian tubes may occasionally become infected and blocked, leading to infertility.

Appetite, loss of

The desire to eat is controlled by cells in a part of the brain called the hypothalamus. In a healthy person, these cells integrate information about the fullness of the digestive system, concentrations of nutrients in the blood, the individual's emotional state and whether food is palatable or not. Depending on the balance of these factors, a person may feel full, comfortable (neither hungry nor full), hungry or have no desire for their food.

Social factors also play an important part in determining when people eat food: the internal controls that register when the stomach is full are often overridden.

CAUSES

Sometimes a loss of appetite is nothing to worry about. It may be caused by a slowing of the growth rate in young people, and in women by decreasing oestrogen levels during the menopause or hormone changes during pregnancy. Loss of appetite may also be an adverse reaction to medication – if you think this could apply to you, check with a doctor.

But a seriously diminished appetite can also be an indication of various diseases and conditions, including:

■ a **kidney** disorder;

■ a **liver** disorder;

■ **cancer**;

■ a viral infection such as infectious mononucleosis (see **Glandular fever**);

■ inadequate levels of cortisone hormone (see **Adrenal glands and disorders**);

■ an underactive **thyroid** gland;

■ vitamin deficiency caused by alcohol abuse, or vitamin B_{12} and folic acid deficiency;

■ stomach inflammation (see **Gastritis** and **Stomach and disorders**);

■ irritation or infection of the digestive tract such as that caused by **food poisoning** (see also **Gastroenteritis** and **Digestive system**);

■ a disorder of the red blood cells (see **Anaemia** and **Blood and disorders**);

■ **stress**, **depression** or **anxiety**;

■ an **eating disorder**.

TREATMENT

If loss of appetite continues for more than a few weeks, seek medical advice for diagnosis and treatment of underlying causes.

What you can do

■ If appetite loss is an acute symptom of food poisoning or of a viral infection lasting only a few days, a diet of plain boiled white rice and plain boiled, cooled water should help.

■ If nausea is one of the acute symptoms, ginger root (or dried ginger powder) in hot water may help. Dried cinnamon in water may help.

■ Where food poisoning with salmonella has occurred, cranberry extract powder dissolved in water helps to remove the micro-organism from the body.

■ If antibiotics have been prescribed to treat appetite loss, a course of a probiotic supplement (containing organisms such as lactobacillus acidophilus and bifidobacteria) together with fructo-oligosaccharides (the growth medium for the probiotic species) can be useful in allowing repopulation of the gastro-intestinal tract with 'healthy' species of bacteria.

SEE ALSO *Diet*

Appetite suppressants

People suffering from **obesity** may find that appetite-suppressant drugs help them to lose weight, but these drugs, which must be prescribed by a doctor, should be used only in conjunction with appropriate changes to **diet**.

Stimulant drugs work within the brain to suppress the appetite. But stimulants (which are similar to amphetamines) can bring about dependence, and there are other serious safety concerns about their use, including possible toxicity. For these reasons, they are used only as a specialist short-term treatment and only for selected patients.

A newer drug, sibutramine, is said to enhance the feeling of being satisfied after eating less food. Rather than being a stimulant, it works in the same way as some **antidepressants**.

Another drug that may aid weight reduction is orlistat (brand name Xenical), which reduces absorption of dietary fat into the body.

Bulking agents such as bran, ispaghula husk, methylcellulose and sterculia offer an alternative to drugs. They work by making the body feel as though it has taken in more food than it actually has.

SEE ALSO *Drugs, medicinal*

Arm and problems

The arm is made up of three long bones: the longest, the humerus, is in the upper arm; the radius and the ulna are in the forearm. The rounded, upper end of the humerus forms a joint with the cup of the shoulder blade and it meets the ulna at the elbow joint. The radius meets the ulna inside the capsule surrounding this joint, and both bones connect with the carpal bones of the wrist joint. The main muscles of the upper arm are the biceps and triceps, which raise (flex) and lower (extend) the forearm. There are two main groups of muscles in the forearm: the wrist and finger extensors, which pull the wrist back and extend the fingers; and the wrist and finger flexors, which pull the hand down and close the grip. The muscles move the bones of the arm, wrist and fingers by means of tendons. Commands for muscle movements are relayed from the brain by the median, ulna and radial nerves.

Blood circulates in the arm through the brachial artery (to the upper arm) and the radial and ulnar arteries (to the forearm).

WHAT CAN GO WRONG

■ **Fractures** of the arm are common; the lower ends of the radius and ulna are the most commonly fractured bones in the body. A blow to the ulna nerve at the 'funny bone' – where the nerve passes over the bottom part of the humerus at the elbow joint – can cause intense discomfort but is unlikely to cause a serious problem.

■ Many common arm problems, such as **arthritis** or **RSI** (repetitive strain injury), involve the joints and muscles. Arthritis and **tendonitis** can affect the elbow and the structures around it (see also **Tennis elbow**), while acute frictional **tenosynovitis** may cause pain in the tendons of the wrist and fingers at the lower end of the forearm.

■ An infection can sometimes develop in one of the arm's bones, generally as a consequence of a serious fracture or of a blood infection (see **Osteomyelitis**).

■ Primary **cancers** only rarely develop in the arm, although secondary cancers, which have spread from elsewhere, sometimes affect the humerus. Benign tumours can affect the arm, although less frequently than they affect the leg. One of them, called a giant-cell tumour (osteoclastoma), may affect the lower end of the radius. Another, made up of cartilage, is known as a chondroma; in the arm this most commonly affects the small bones of the hands but it can also occur in the humerus.

■ Pain in the arm can be the result of a problem elsewhere, such as in the cervical spine, brachial

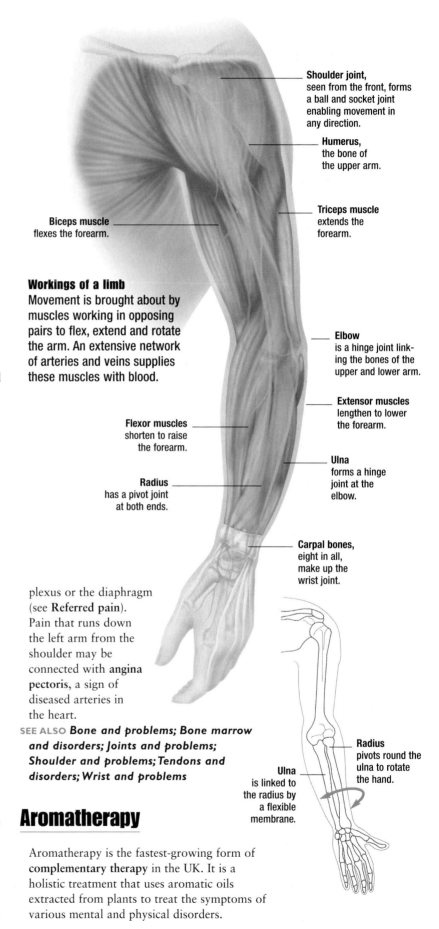

Shoulder joint, seen from the front, forms a ball and socket joint enabling movement in any direction.

Humerus, the bone of the upper arm.

Triceps muscle extends the forearm.

Biceps muscle flexes the forearm.

Elbow is a hinge joint linking the bones of the upper and lower arm.

Extensor muscles lengthen to lower the forearm.

Ulna forms a hinge joint at the elbow.

Carpal bones, eight in all, make up the wrist joint.

Radius pivots round the ulna to rotate the hand.

Ulna is linked to the radius by a flexible membrane.

Workings of a limb
Movement is brought about by muscles working in opposing pairs to flex, extend and rotate the arm. An extensive network of arteries and veins supplies these muscles with blood.

Flexor muscles shorten to raise the forearm.

Radius has a pivot joint at both ends.

plexus or the diaphragm (see **Referred pain**). Pain that runs down the left arm from the shoulder may be connected with **angina pectoris**, a sign of diseased arteries in the heart.

SEE ALSO *Bone and problems; Bone marrow and disorders; Joints and problems; Shoulder and problems; Tendons and disorders; Wrist and problems*

Aromatherapy

Aromatherapy is the fastest-growing form of **complementary therapy** in the UK. It is a holistic treatment that uses aromatic oils extracted from plants to treat the symptoms of various mental and physical disorders.

During an aromatherapy massage session, one or more aromatic oils are diluted in a carrier oil and smoothed into the skin. Aromatherapy oils (known as essential oils) can also be inhaled, added to bath water or used in a compress.

There have been several **clinical trials** on aromatherapy. In a survey of 8000 women in childbirth midwives at Oxford's John Radcliffe Hospital found that a lavender-oil massage reduced the need for drug-based pain relief in labour by 60 per cent.

HOW IT CAN HELP

Aromatherapy can help to promote relaxation and general well-being. It is also used to treat specific problems and disorders such as:

■ **stress** or anxiety-related conditions, including heart and digestive problems;

■ premenstrual syndrome, symptoms of the menopause and other hormone-related disorders affecting women;

■ sleeping difficulties.

THE ORTHODOX VIEW

Since aromatherapy does not interfere with orthodox medical treatments, an increasing number of NHS staff now use it as part of an integrated care programme in the treatment of patients suffering from cancer, AIDS or heart problems. However, many doctors view it as no more than a relaxing therapy.

WHAT'S INVOLVED

An aromatherapist should take a medical history, listen to why you have come, then choose the oils. A session usually lasts 1–1½ hrs.

A specific problem may require weekly treatments for many weeks, or you may choose to have a monthly session as a treat. After an aromatherapy massage, most people feel relaxed.

Side effects may include skin irritation, an allergic reaction or an episode of dizziness. Report any signs of these to your therapist before the next treatment.

PRECAUTIONS

■ Aromatherapy is not suitable for people with epilepsy; some oils, including cinnamon, ginger, rosemary and thyme, should be avoided by people suffering from high blood pressure.

■ Apart from tea tree and lavender, oils should not be applied neat to the skin. No oils should be used on broken skin.

■ Certain oils should be avoided in pregnancy. These include basil, black pepper, cinnamon, clary sage, clove, eucalyptus, fennel, hyssop, juniper, thyme, marjoram, rosemary and sage.

■ Do not take an oil by mouth unless advised to do so by a medically trained aromatherapist.

SELF-HELP

Aromatherapy oils are available from health-food shops and pharmacies. If you are, or may be, pregnant, or if you have a pre-existing

Essential oils

The properties of essential oils produce a range of effects on the body and mind.

OIL	EFFECT
Bergamot	Refreshing and uplifting
Black pepper	Stimulates appetite
Camomile	Promotes peaceful sleep
Cedarwood	Calming; diminishes fear
Clary sage	Calming and reassuring
Eucalyptus	Stimulating and restorative
Jasmine	Encourages self-confidence
Lavender	Soothing; reduces anxiety
Lemon	Invigorating; clarifies thought
Neroli	Relieves nervous tension
Peppermint	Stimulating and reviving
Pine	Stimulating and refreshing
Rose	Calming and uplifting
Rosemary	Invigorating
Sandalwood	Relaxing and sensual
Tea tree	Antifungal and antiseptic
Ylang Ylang	Relieves anxiety and frustration

health condition, consult an aromatherapist before using oils at home. Similarly, seek advice from a therapist before treating children.

CONTACT **Aromatherapy Consortium** PO Box 6522, Desborough, Kettering, Northants NN14 2YX 0870 774 3477 (www.aromatherapy-regulation.org.uk)

Arrhythmia

Arrhythmia is any condition in which there is an abnormality in the electrical impulse through the heart, which may cause the heart to beat too fast, too slowly, or irregularly. The cause may be underlying heart disease, medical conditions such as **thyroid** disease, or external forces such as **stress**, drugs, alcohol, electric shock or extremes of temperature.

The heart rate may be too rapid or too uncoordinated to allow the heart to fill up properly between beats, or it may be too slow to pump blood effectively round the body.

Arrhythmias can cause fatigue, low blood pressure (hypotension), faintness, breathlessness or chest pain. Drugs, heart surgery, electric shock treatment (defibrillation) or a **pacemaker** may be needed to counteract these effects, as well as treatment of the underlying cause.

Arteries and disorders

As a whole, our arteries constitute a branching system of tubes that carries blood to every tissue in the body. The main arterial 'tree' transports oxygenated blood; the much smaller pulmonary artery picks up blood that has returned to the heart, taking it to the lungs to collect more oxygen.

The **aorta** is the trunk of the arterial tree. Smaller arteries branch off and subdivide until they become arterioles, which are less than 0.1mm in diameter and flow into the blood vessels (capillaries) that supply individual cells. Arterioles receive their own supply of oxygen from the blood they carry; larger arteries are supplied from outside by small arterial 'twigs'.

Muscles in the artery walls contract or relax to control the diameter of the arteries and regulate the blood flow. Sometimes this muscle layer or the artery lining may become stiff or damaged and the arteries may narrow, causing conditions such as aneurysm, arteriosclerosis and arteritis.

Arterial aneurysm

Arterial **aneurysm** is a condition in which weakness, then a swelling, develops in an arterial wall. The aorta is most commonly affected, but aneurysms can affect arteries supplying the brain, limbs or internal organs. The main cause is arteriosclerosis, but infection, sudden physical injury, surgery or congenital abnormalities can also trigger an aneurysm.

SYMPTOMS

There may be no symptoms, but seek medical help urgently if you suffer signs of leaking or rupture (bursting) of the artery, such as collapse and shock, or a tearing pain in the chest, abdomen or back. Medical advice should also be sought if you experience:
- painless swelling in the abdomen, neck, arm or leg, which pulses in time to the heartbeat;
- symptoms due to pressure such as abdominal pain, difficulty in swallowing or headaches.

TREATMENT

A leaking aneurysm is a life-threatening condition that requires emergency hospital admission. In less urgent cases, a doctor may arrange tests and set up monitoring procedures.

What a doctor may do
- Check for and, if necessary, treat diabetes, hypertension or raised **cholesterol**.
- Examine the artery by ultrasound, magnetic resonance imaging (MRI) or angiography.
- Monitor the growth of an aneurysm using ultrasound every 6–12 months. Surgery may be needed if an abdominal aortic aneurysm grows larger than 5.5cm (2in) in diameter.

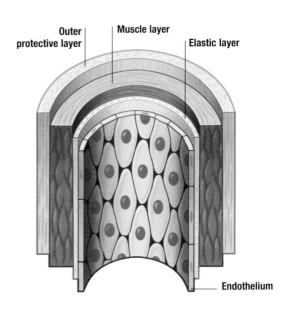

Outer protective layer · Muscle layer · Elastic layer · Endothelium

▲ **Inside a healthy artery**
An artery's inner lining, or endothelium, is enclosed by an elastic layer, a smooth muscle layer (which regulates blood flow) and an outer protective layer.

- Advise on changes to a patient's lifestyle that should reduce the risk of further damage.

Surgical options
Surgery can take one of several forms.
- The diseased section of artery may be bypassed using a section of vein or synthetic tubing.
- A polyester fibre lining tube may be inserted into the artery to provide a new 'inner tube'. In the case of an abdominal aortic aneurysm, a Y-shaped tube is used where the aorta divides into the iliac arteries.
- An endarterectomy may be performed to correct an abdominal aortic aneurysm. This involves reconstruction of the aorto-iliac segment of artery after removal of the diseased section and most of the artery lining.

COMPLICATIONS

The most serious risk posed by an aneurysm is rupture. Sometimes a rupture is incomplete and occurs between the inner and outer layers of the arterial wall. Another possible complication is arterial thrombosis.

PREVENTION

Adopting a healthier lifestyle reduces the chance of further damage (see arteriosclerosis, below).

Abdominal aortic aneurysm affects up to 10,000 people a year in the UK, mostly men over the age of 60. Those at particular risk should have regular ultrasound screening. They include people with a father or brother who has suffered aortic aneurysm, arteriosclerosis, hypertension or ischaemic heart disease.

Arterial thrombosis

Arterial thrombosis is a condition in which an artery becomes blocked, cutting off the blood supply to body organs or tissues. The affected organ or tissue may become damaged or even die. Thrombosis occurs if the blood flows too slowly or clots too easily, and is often the final result of narrowing and hardening of the artery.

Arteriosclerosis

Arteriosclerosis – also known as or atherosclerosis – develops over many years. It is a significant cause of heart attacks, strokes and circulatory and memory problems.

As the condition evolves, fatty streaks appear on the artery linings and progress to become fibrous cholesterol-containing plaques (raised circular areas), reducing the diameter of the arteries. The artery walls gradually stiffen – a process called hardening of the arteries – and organs or limbs can become starved of oxygen and other nutrients, leading to permanent damage. Weak points (aneurysms) or blockages (thromboses) may also develop. If the arteries in the neck are arteriosclerotic, the oxygen supply to the brain may be affected, especially when the neck is turned, leading to dizziness.

SYMPTOMS

Arteriosclerosis affects most people by late middle-age, but it has no symptoms until complications such as angina or stroke develop.

TREATMENT

If you consult a doctor about the condition, your **blood pressure** will be checked and the levels of cholesterol and sugar in your blood will be measured. Drugs may be prescribed to reduce blood pressure or levels of cholesterol or blood sugar. You may also be given advice about losing weight, restricting alcohol intake, adopting a healthier diet and stopping smoking.

What you can do

Complications associated with arteriosclerosis can be delayed or prevented by making changes to your lifestyle that will reduce health risks. These may include:

- losing weight – see **Body Mass Index (BMI)**;
- stopping smoking;
- restricting alcohol consumption to 21–28 units per week for men and 14–21 for women;
- walking briskly for at least 20 minutes five times a week;
- eating a low-fat diet that includes cholesterol-lowering foods;
- lowering stress levels;
- having regular blood pressure checks.

Complementary therapies

Fenugreek seeds are believed to lower the levels of cholesterol and sugar in the blood, thereby enhancing good circulation.

Factfile

Arteriosclerosis – who is at risk?

Arteriosclerosis develops over a number of years but there are certain factors that are known to increase the risk of developing the disease.

- Being a man.
- Being of Asian origin.
- Having a parent or sibling who developed coronary heart disease before the age of 55.
- Being a smoker.
- Having a diet high in cholesterol and saturated fats, and low in fresh fruit, vegetables and fibre.
- Having high blood cholesterol levels.
- Suffering from hypertension.
- Suffering from diabetes mellitus.
- Being severely obese.
- Having high blood levels of particular proteins: lipoprotein, fibrinogen or homocysteine.

▲ **Narrowing and stiffening of an artery** If an artery's inner wall is damaged, fats, heavy metals, clotting agents and blood cells all stick to the affected area. The immune system tries to heal the wound and to form a cap of fibrous material, or plaque. Buildup of plaque narrows the artery.

Arteriovenous fistula

Arteriovenous fistula is a disorder in which an artery drains directly into a vein. The abnormal connection (fistula) causes swollen veins and may deprive the rest of the artery of blood, reducing oxygen supply. If excessive blood is diverted through the fistula, heart failure can develop and the artery may need to be blocked using a tiny coil or plug. The condition may be congenital or the result of an injury or disease.

Arteritis

Arteritis is a condition in which the muscle wall of one or more arteries becomes inflamed, causing narrowing and reduced blood flow. Large, medium or small arteries may be affected. Symptoms include pain and tenderness of the affected skin region – the fingers, for example – or internal organ such as the aorta.

The cause is often unclear, although damage to the artery's own blood supply may be to blame. Arteritis is sometimes linked with diseases such as rheumatoid arthritis or immune system malfunction – in polyarteritis nodosa, for instance. In people with polyarteritis nodosa, the medium-sized arteries become inflamed, reducing blood supply and causing damage to the organs; symptoms include abdominal and testicular pain, chest pain, breathing difficulty or tender lumps under the skin, depending on which organs are affected.

In temporal arteritis, which affects older people, arteries in the scalp become inflamed, causing headaches and scalp tenderness; this can spread to retinal arteries, causing blindness if the condition is not treated.

Treatment of arteritis with anti-inflammatory drugs including steroids is often successful, but lifestyle changes, especially stopping **smoking**, are important in preventing further artery damage. Damaged organs such as the heart or kidney may require additional treatment.

Peripheral arterial disease

In peripheral arterial disease the blood supply to a limb or tissue is reduced or cut off, leading to blood and oxygen shortage (ischaemia). It is commonly caused by a gradual narrowing of the artery. Total blockage may suddenly occur in the form of arterial thrombosis, or a blood clot may break off and travel to block another artery (embolism). Ischaemia may also develop after sudden physical injury, including surgery.

SYMPTOMS

■ A cramp-like pain, which is worse when oxygen demands are high but disappears after rest – for example, in the calf muscles on walking. Pain at rest indicates severe ischaemia.
■ Cold, pale feet or toes that turn blue.
■ Gradual or sudden tissue damage in the legs (leg ulcers, gangrene), heart (angina), brain (stroke) or internal organs.
■ Sudden severe pain in an arm or leg, which turns cold and white.
■ Severe pain in the chest, abdomen or back.

TREATMENT

If you have any of the above symptoms, consult a doctor; if pain is sudden and severe, seek medical advice urgently. If arterial aneurysm, thrombosis, embolism or severe ischaemia is suspected, you will need surgery or treatment to break up clots. In less urgent cases, a doctor may arrange tests and monitoring procedures.

What a doctor may do
■ Check for and, if necessary, treat diabetes, hypertension or raised cholesterol.
■ Measure the arterial pressure in your legs using Doppler ultrasound.

■ Refer you for ultrasound, angiography or magnetic resonance imaging (MRI).
■ Advise you on beneficial lifestyle changes.
■ Prescribe a daily dose of 75mg aspirin.

Surgical options
Surgery may take one of several forms, such as:
■ angioplasty – artery widening or repair;
■ grafting – replacement of diseased section of leg artery with part of another artery or vein;
■ sympathectomy – keyhole surgery or chemical injection that severs the nerves in the back that control leg artery diameter;
■ amputation of foot or leg if gangrene occurs.

COMPLICATIONS

Poor oxygen supply to the legs may lead to leg ulcers. In more serious cases there is a risk of gangrene – and of failure of part or all of a body organ due to lack of oxygen.

PREVENTION

The best way to prevent peripheral arterial disease is to adopt a healthier lifestyle. Avoid dehydration and prolonged sitting or kneeling, which encourage blood clotting.

Raynaud's syndrome

Raynaud's syndrome is a condition in which spasm of small arteries (arterioles), usually in the fingers, produces colour changes – paleness followed by blueness then redness – as well as numbness and sometimes pain.

Raynaud's syndrome may occur as a result of scleroderma, an autoimmune disease causing the skin to thicken, swell and scar on the hands and feet, which become stiff, tight and shiny; ulceration and even gangrene may develop.

Treatment consists of wearing warm or artificially heated gloves and clothing. Drugs such as nifedipine are used to dilate the arterioles. As in all arterial diseases, it is important to stop smoking.

Takayasu's disease

Takayasu's disease is a condition of unknown cause in which inflammation and thrombosis in the aorta and other arteries lead to reduced pulses in the limbs, dizziness, raised blood pressure and aortic and other aneurysms. It is also known as 'pulseless disease' and is treated with corticosteroids and arterial surgery.

CONTACT **British Vascular Foundation**
Fides House, 10 Chertsey Road, Woking, Surrey GU21 5AB, fax (01483) 726522 (www.bvf.org.uk)
Raynaud's and Scleroderma Association
112 Crewe Road, Alsager, Cheshire ST7 2JA (01270) 872776 (www.raynauds.org.uk)
The Royal Free Hospital Vascular Unit
(www.freevas.demon.co.uk)

Arthritis

Seven million people in the UK suffer from one of the many forms of arthritis, which cause pain, stiffness, swelling and loss of mobility in affected joints. Fortunately, treatments are becoming more effective.

Although arthritis is widespread – about one-fifth of visits to doctors in the UK are arthritis-related – there is an increasingly optimistic outlook for sufferers. Arthritic disease takes many forms, and varies enormously in the severity of its symptoms. But the treatments to alleviate it are becoming ever more effective. For example, lost mobility can now be restored by replacing damaged joints with artificial ones made from alloys of steel and plastics that do not react to the body's tissues or provoke rejection by the immune system.

Shoulders, elbows, hips and knees can all be successfully replaced. Replacement of finger joints in people who were previously unable to open their hands has proved so effective that in some cases, after recovering from surgery, they are able to thread needles.

RHEUMATOID AND OSTEOARTHRITIS

Two widespread forms of arthritis, rheumatoid arthritis and osteoarthritis, are chronic disorders that are unlikely to go away once established – as opposed to some other types, such as reactive arthritis, which do not persist and can go away on their own. Both rheumatoid and osteoarthritis, typically, have 'flare-ups', interrupted by periods of remission that bring spontaneous relief from pain.

Rheumatoid arthritis, which affects about one in 150 people in the UK, is a painful, progressive, inflammatory condition. Joints in the fingers, wrists, knees and shoulders are the most likely to become inflamed. Rheumatoid arthritis can also cause skin lumps (nodules) and damage to the lungs and eyes.

The first signs of the disease are joint pains and stiffness and an under-the-weather feeling, beginning usually between the ages of 30 and 50, although it can strike at any time of life.

Inflammation starts in the lining of the joint (synovium), but it often leads on to damage to the surrounding bones – which is why it is essential to begin treatment early. Treatment focuses on controlling inflammation, alleviating pain and reducing complications. It may involve anti-inflammatory drugs, physiotherapy, exercise and in some cases joint-replacement surgery.

The cause of rheumatoid arthritis is unknown, but it is thought that the body's immune system turns against the tissue and bone in the joint and starts to attack them. As the disease sometimes run in families, it may have a genetic element (see **Genetics and genetic disorders**).

By contrast, osteoarthritis is a degenerative condition with a 'wear-and-tear' element – the protective, shock-absorbing cartilage space

Arthritis in the knee joint

Rheumatoid and osteoarthritis can affect any joint, but osteoarthritis is commoner in the knee.

Rheumatoid arthritis is characterized by an inflammation that starts in the synovial membrane lining the joint cavity, but soon progresses to cause damage to the surrounding bones.

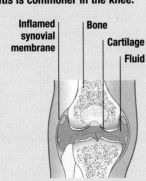

Inflamed synovial membrane | Bone | Cartilage | Fluid

Osteoarthritis involves damage to the cartilage-covered bone surfaces in a joint that act as shock absorbers; extra bone forms at the joint edges.

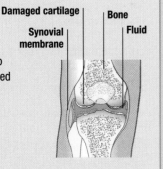

Damaged cartilage | Synovial membrane | Bone | Fluid

▲ **Joint distortion**
This X-ray of a hand affected by rheumatoid arthritis shows the distortion of the knuckle bones caused by inflammation of the joints.

Different types of arthritic disease

X-rays and MRI scans can confirm a diagnosis of arthritis. Blood tests are used to identify specific conditions such as rheumatoid arthritis.

DISORDER	DISTINGUISHING FEATURES
Inflammatory types such as rheumatoid arthritis, septic arthritis and gout	The joint lining becomes inflamed. This can damage the surface of the joint and underlying bone
Rheumatoid arthritis	A chronic (recurring) autoimmune disease
Reactive arthritis	Develops after viral or bacterial infection has occurred somewhere else in the body
Septic arthritis	Viral, bacterial or fungal infection at joint site. Treated with intravenous antibiotics
Gout	Excess uric acid causes inflammation in toe joint. An inherited condition that comes and goes
Pseudogout	Calcium crystals form, usually on the knee
Ankylosing spondylitis	Inflammation and fusing of lower vertebrae in spine
Psoriatic arthritis	Associated with psoriasis or colitis
Connective tissue diseases	Include systemic lupus erythematosus
Cervical spondylosis	Spurs of bone form on the neck vertebrae
Polyarteritis nodosa	Rare form of vasculitis, inflammation of medium and small arteries, with impaired circulation. Cause unknown
Osteoarthritis	The cartilage becomes thinner and damaged and extra bone forms at the edges of the joint. Can occur in any joint. Chronic. Immune system not involved.

There are more than 2 million people with osteoarthritis in the UK. More women than men suffer from the disease.

between the bones of the joints wears away with age, and new spurs of bone often form at the edges of the joint. Starting from mid-life, osteoarthritis affects mainly the hip, knees, spine and fingers, but can occur in any joint. Abnormal stress, injury to a joint, or obesity, which places extra weight on a joint, may cause the disease to develop.

In more than 50 per cent of osteoarthritis cases, there is remission of pain for many years after an initial painful period.

OTHER FORMS OF ARTHRITIS

There are several other common inflammatory types of the disease, which include:
■ reactive arthritis, which can develop after a viral or bacterial infection somewhere else in the body;
■ septic arthritis, where there is a viral, bacterial or fungal infection at a joint site;
■ gout, where an excess of uric acid leads to inflammation in the toe joint, for example.

These varieties of arthritis strike intermittently. Chronic types include connective tissue diseases such as systemic lupus erythematosus, and ankylosing spondylitis, involving inflammation and fusing of the lower vertebrae in the spine.

DIAGNOSING ARTHRITIS

Differing symptoms offer clues for distinguishing between one form of arthritis and another. A general feeling of malaise and severe flare-ups are pointers to rheumatoid arthritis, for example.

If an arthritic condition is suspected, doctors can use X-rays and magnetic resonance imaging (MRI) scans to confirm a diagnosis. Blood tests are carried out to show up a specific condition and to identify or eliminate other diseases.

Management of any chronic arthritic disease is a team job involving GPs, rheumatologists, orthopaedic surgeons, physiotherapists and occupational therapists.

TREATMENT

If you have pain, swelling or stiffness that continues for more than six weeks, consult a doctor and ask to be referred to a rheumatologist.

Most arthritic diseases can be effectively controlled and alleviated by modern treatment. As both severity of symptoms and symptoms themselves vary greatly from person to person, treatment needs to be tailored to each individual.

Appropriate drugs and **complementary therapies** combined with **physiotherapy** to help improve movement and instruction on how to protect the joints can often restore sufferers to full lives and minimize their discomfort. If there is severe joint damage and resultant disability, surgery may prove necessary to replace the damaged joint.

Arthritis drugs

A wide range of drugs is used to treat the symptoms and slow progression of arthritic diseases (see **Drugs, medicinal**).
■ Analgesics such as paracetamol reduce pain.
■ Non-steroidal anti-inflammatory drugs (NSAIDs) reduce swelling and stiffness, and alleviate pain. But they can also irritate the stomach lining so no one should take NSAIDs for more than three days unless under medical supervision. Taking NSAIDs over a long period of time can lead to chronic bleeding ulcers, which can prove fatal in a small number of cases.
■ Used early in the development of rheumatoid arthritis, some drugs can slow the progression of the condition. Anti-rheumatic drugs such as the immunosuppressant methotrexate and the anti-inflammatory sulfasalazine can be used on

a long-term basis. Gold salts, penicillamine and choroquine may work by suppressing the disease process itself.

■ Steroids are powerful anti-inflammatory agents that can be injected or taken in tablet form.

Breakthrough treatments

■ People with rheumatoid arthritis have an excessive amount of the protein TNF (tumour necrosis factor) in their blood and joints. Drugs are available to block the action of TNF, reducing inflammation. Such immunosuppressive drugs are prescribed when standard treatments have not been effective.

■ A new generation of NSAIDs have a stronger anti-inflammatory effect than their predecessors, but are less likely to cause intestinal irritation. Hyaluronic acid and derivatives are new non-steroidal drugs that, when injected into the knee joint, temporarily reduce pain and inflammation.

■ Clinical trials are underway to investigate a drug regime that targets the B-cells – the white blood cells that can accidentally make antibodies that destroy healthy tissue.

Complementary therapies

■ The food supplements glucosamine sulphate and fish oil have been proven to have mild anti-inflammatory effects.

■ Warmth may ease pain in osteoarthritic fingers. A cold compress may ease an inflamed joint.

■ For rheumatoid arthritis, try taking two teaspoons of apple cider vinegar in some hot water, twice a day. This can be sweetened with honey to taste, if preferred.

ARTHRITIS IN CHILDREN

One child in 1000 has arthritis. The condition occurs most often at ages 1–4 years, and again at 10–13 years. To counter confusion of names and various presentations of arthritic disease in children, the accepted term in the UK for childhood arthritis is now 'juvenile idiopathic arthritis' ('idiopathic' means 'without clear external cause').

Symptoms are varied and can be confused with other conditions – for example, initially there may be a fever, swollen glands and general aching. Seek out full investigation and careful diagnosis. Treatment involves removal of fluid from the affected joints, drugs such as anti-inflammatories or steroid injections. Regular, gentle exercise often helps to keep joints flexible.

CONTACT **Arthritis Research Campaign** Copeman House, St Mary's Court, St Mary's Gate, Chesterfield, Derbyshire S41 7TD 0870 850 5000 (www.arc.org.uk) **Arthritis Care** 18 Stephenson Way, London NW1 2HD; helpline 0808 800 4050 noon–4pm Mon–Fri; Under-25s (The Source) 0808 808 2000 10am–2pm Mon–Fri (www.arthritiscare.org.uk)

> While the pain of rheumatoid arthritis tends to be worst in the morning, the pain of osteoarthritis gets worse as the day goes on.

Living with arthritis

It helps to be positive about arthritis and it is vital to realize that there are many ways in which you can help yourself.

■ Do not let the condition prevent you doing the things you want to do.

■ Exercise keeps bones strong, and muscles toned, and keeping active is good for general health. It is important to keep joints moving so that they do not stiffen up.

■ Eat a healthy, balanced diet with plenty of fruit, fibre and vegetables. Reduce meat consumption and replace animal fats with olive oil and fish oils.

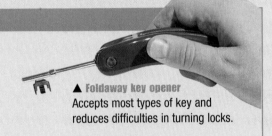

▲ **Foldaway key opener** Accepts most types of key and reduces difficulties in turning locks.

There are many gadgets available that can make life easier for arthritis sufferers.

■ Twister openers that grip the tops of bottle and jars.

■ Handiplugs, enabling an easy grip on electrical plugs.

■ Tap turner that adapts to most modern tap designs and allows the tap to be turned on and off.

■ Foldaway key opener that provides a more substantial handle to grasp when turning keys in locks.

■ Ultra-lightweight Handi-Reacher to help with everything from drawing curtains and dressing, to picking up anything effortlessly.

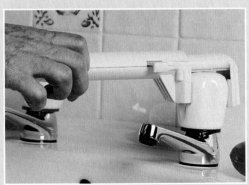

◀ **Tap turner** The easy-fit design clips over modern tap fittings.

Arthroplasty

An arthroplasty is an operation in which a joint is repaired or replaced to improve its function. One of the most common types of arthroplasty is a hip-joint replacement, in which the hip joint (usually damaged by **arthritis**) is replaced with a new artificial joint.

Artificial insemination

Artificial insemination is a fertility technique in which semen is introduced into the cervix using a syringe in order for the woman to conceive. In Artificial Insemination by Donor (AID), the semen is provided by an anonymous donor.
SEE ALSO *Infertility*

Artificial respiration

Artificial respiration, also known as the kiss of life, is an emergency procedure used in first aid to ventilate the lungs of a person who has stopped breathing (when drowning or unconscious, for example). Respiration, or breathing, is the natural process of transporting oxygen and carbon dioxide to and from the lungs. If someone stops breathing, the oxygen level in the blood drops quickly. Within six minutes brain damage will take place and death will not be far off. Artificial respiration may take the form of mouth-to-mouth or mouth-to-nose resuscitation. The person giving artificial respiration makes regular out breathes into the patient's mouth or nose so that the lungs are inflated and continues until breathing returns.
SEE ALSO *FIRST AID; Respiratory system*

Artificial ventilation

The medical process of mechanical support for breathing is called artificial ventilation. It may also be referred to as artificial respiration.

Artificial ventilation is used in hospitals whenever respiratory failure occurs or is likely to occur – for example, during an operation or in an emergency. Ventilators can either assist breathing or control it entirely. They work by forcing air into the lungs to allow the oxygen exchange process to take place.

Ventilators are designed to mimic the natural process of breathing as closely as possible, but since they deliver oxygen at high pressure they sometimes cause damage to the lungs or ears.
SEE ALSO *Lungs and disorders; Respiratory system*

Asbestosis

Asbestosis is a lung disease caused by inhaling asbestos fibres. It is characterized by scarring of the lung tissue. The main symptoms are shortness of breath, a persistent cough and, less commonly, chest pains. The onset of symptoms can occur between 10 and 40 years after exposure to asbestos. People with asbestosis are more at risk of developing lung cancers and up to 55 times more at risk if they also smoke.

The use of asbestos was regulated in the UK in the early 1970s, but because the symptoms take so many years to develop some 3500 people a year are still dying of asbestosis.
SEE ALSO *Lungs and disorders; Occupational health*

Ascites

Ascites is an abnormal buildup of fluid in the abdominal cavity causing swelling and discomfort. Sufferers may feel short of breath, lose their appetite or regurgitate their food. The most common cause of ascites is cirrhosis of the liver, but other causes include heart failure, kidney disease, pancreatic disease, tuberculosis and some cancers.

To diagnose ascites, a doctor will remove some of the fluid with a needle and send it for analysis or recommend an **ultrasound** scan. Treatment often includes bed rest and a low-salt diet. Diuretics, which make the kidneys excrete more fluid in the urine, can also be used. Ascites sufferers who have liver disease must not drink alcohol.
SEE ALSO *Abdominal pain*

Aseptic technique

The term 'aseptic technique' covers the various procedures involved in ensuring an infection-free environment suitable for medical practice. It includes regular handwashing with antiseptic soap and the use of sterile disposable equipment and implements.

Asperger's syndrome

Asperger's syndrome is a type of **autism** in which social intelligence is severely impaired. People with this condition show normal or even exceptional intelligence in areas that do not involve social interaction. However, they lack 'theory of mind' – the ability to know intuitively what is going on in another person's thoughts – and tend to be very literal-minded. As a result, Asperger's sufferers are very poor at recognizing signs of emotion, which makes them appear insensitive.

In common with other forms of autism, Asperger's syndrome is marked by a rigid adherence to routine and attention to detail. People with Asperger's are therefore often very good at repetitive tasks requiring high accuracy.

Aspergillosis

Aspergillosis is an infection of the lungs and airways caused by aspergillus, a fungus that grows on decaying vegetation. While harmless to healthy people, aspergillus may worsen the symptoms of people with **asthma**. It may also lead to inflammation of the lungs and recurrent chest infections.

Aspergillosis can cause a fungus ball to form in people whose lungs have been damaged by tuberculosis, causing them to cough up blood. The disease can be fatal in people with impaired immune systems and those who have undergone transplant operations.

Aspergillosis can be diagnosed by skin or blood tests. It is treated by antifungal drugs and, where appropriate, anti-asthma drugs.

Aspermia, Azoospermia

Aspermia is a rare condition in which no semen is produced. It is believed to affect around 1 in 1000 men in the UK. Azoospermia, affecting about 1 in 200 men, is a condition where semen is produced but very little or no sperm. The causes of both may be hormonal, genetic or physical. Some cancer treatments may cause temporary aspermia. Azoospermia is the desired result in a vasectomy (see **Sterilization**).

More common is oligospermia, a condition where the ejaculate contains fewer sperm than normal (see **Reproductive system**).

While many cases of aspermia or azoospermia are difficult to treat, if any sperm is present, a man may be helped to father a child, using intracytoplasmic sperm injection (ICSI) or in vitro fertilization.

Asphyxia

Asphyxia, or suffocation, is a life-threatening condition in which inhaled oxygen fails to reach the tissues of the body as a result of damage to or obstruction of any part of the respiratory system, including oxygen carried by blood. The

causes include heart failure, choking, drowning, electric shock and breathing poisonous gas. Oxygen supplies in the body run out within a few minutes if breathing is stopped. If cells in the body, particularly those in the brain and heart, are starved of oxygen, it can lead to unconsciousness and death.

SEE ALSO *Anoxia; Artificial respiration; FIRST AID*

Aspiration

Aspiration is a procedure for withdrawing fluids, gases, debris or harmful material from the body. It is done using a machine called an aspirator, which works by suction.

SEE ALSO *Breathing difficulties; Bronchopneumonia*

Aspirin

Aspirin, or acetylsalicylic acid, is a painkilling (analgesic) drug. Introduced in Germany in 1899, Aspirin was originally the trade name, but now it is used as the generic, or common, name. It was developed from the natural painkiller and fever-lowering drug salicylic acid, found in meadowsweet, willow and other plants. The name aspirin references the latin for meadowsweet (*Spiraeae ulmania*).

Aspirin is now made entirely synthetically, and is sold in enormous quantities. It is used to treat mild to moderate pain, reduce fever and to reduce inflammation in rheumatic conditions.

More recently, aspirin taken at low doses on a long-term basis has been used as an antiplatelet drug in people at risk from **arterial thrombosis**. It helps to prevent blood platelets from sticking together, so inhibiting the formation of clots.

GENERAL ADVICE

- In tablet form, standard aspirin irritates the stomach lining and can cause bleeding and ulcers, so it is preferable to take the drug in soluble form. Coated preparations – which do not release the aspirin until it reaches the small intestine – are a good alternative.
- People with peptic ulcers or indigestion, or those who are anaemic or hypersensitive to salicylates, should not take aspirin.
- **Paracetamol** rather than aspirin is used for pain relief and for reducing fever in children aged under 16 years and for pregnant or breastfeeding women, because of a possible link between aspirin and the rare but serious disorder Reye's syndrome.
- Aspirin can provoke **asthma** attacks in some people.

SEE ALSO *Drugs, medicinal*

▲ **A better pill**
Soluble aspirin dissolved in water is absorbed into the body more quickly than non-soluble aspirin tablets.

Asthma

Asthma may occur at any age and vary in severity. Some people have infrequent attacks and feel fine in between them; others have to take drugs daily, usually by inhalation, to suppress symptoms.

Asthma attacks can make people feel as if they are suffocating. As they struggle to draw breath through narrowed airways in their lungs, they inhale in short gasps and exhale in long, noisy wheezes. The lower ribcage may contract sharply on inhaled breaths, and the pulse races; in a severe attack, the sufferer's lips may turn blue from loss of oxygen.

Asthma is a condition in which the lining of the airways supplying the lungs swells, restricting air flow and making it hard to breathe. During an attack the airways become narrower; often sticky mucus or phlegm is produced. Sufferers have hypersensitive airways, which are almost always red and slightly inflamed. This means that their lungs are vulnerable to any of a wide range of irritants, including pollen, feathered and furred animals (particularly cats), aspirin and some other drugs, the droppings of house-dust mites, changes in temperature (for example, breathing in very cold air) and cigarette smoke. Some attacks are triggered by non-environmental factors such as respiratory infections, stress, anxiety or exercise.

A GROWING PROBLEM

An estimated 150 million people worldwide suffer from asthma, and every year asthma and other respiratory diseases are becoming more common globally. There are many theories about why this is happening, but none is free of controversy.

The tendency to develop allergic conditions, such as **hay fever**, allergic asthma and **eczema**, often runs in families. If one or both parents suffer from asthma, hay fever or eczema, the chance of their children developing one of these conditions is higher. Scientists are searching for a genetic link in the hope of developing gene therapy to treat the condition.

Common asthma triggers include viral infections, allergies, irritants and exercise. A third of children who suffer from asthma improve during their teenage years, and have fewer symptoms in adult life.

Among new advances in combating asthma is a preventive injection which is undergoing clinical trials and is expected to be licensed in 2005. It is designed to be given every two to four weeks and take the place of existing drug treatments. The drug contains an **antibody** that can knock out the proteins which trigger allergic asthma attacks.

TREATMENT

Once asthma has been diagnosed, you are likely to be prescribed drugs to prevent or relieve asthma attacks. These are called preventers or relievers (see Drug treatments for asthma, right).

If you continue to have frequent attacks in spite of using an inhaler regularly, the doctor may prescribe additional tablets to be taken orally – for example, a short course of **steroid** tablets.

Medical terms

The peak-flow meter measures how fast and how hard you can exhale air from your lungs. This is an indication of how well controlled your asthma is – you cannot blow hard when your airways are inflamed. Your peak-flow reading, when compared with levels set by your doctor or with previous readings, can often predict an asthma attack, even a day or two in advance.

Self-help
Action in an attack

The symptoms of asthma are wheezing or whistling in the chest, shortness of breath, a tight feeling in the chest and coughing (dry or with mucus). Consult a doctor if you have any of these symptoms or if your sleep is being disturbed because of breathing difficulties or coughing. If you have an attack, take the following steps:

- Take two puffs of your reliever inhaler immediately.

- Try to stay calm and relaxed.

- Sit in a position you find comfortable.

- Try to slow your breathing down.

- Call a doctor or ambulance if the inhaler has no effect after five to ten minutes, and keep using your inhaler every few minutes until help arrives.

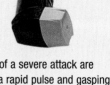

Emergency Symptoms of a severe attack are blue lips, clammy skin, a rapid pulse and gasping for breath. Severe attacks require emergency medical attention.

Drug treatments for asthma

Most people with asthma breathe in the medication they need using an inhaler. Two main types of drugs are taken using inhalers: preventers and relievers.

People use **relievers**, which usually come in blue inhalers, when they are suffering an asthma attack. Relievers relax the muscles surrounding the airways – the drugs should start to ease your breathing in a few minutes and the relief should last up to four hours. **Preventers** make the airways less sensitive, reducing the chance of symptoms developing. Preventers should be used every day, usually once in the morning and once in the evening, even if you are feeling well. They generally come in white, brown, orange or red inhalers.

Some people use **spacers** when taking their asthma medication with inhalers. Spacers are large plastic containers with a mouthpiece at one end and a connection to the inhaler at the other. You can release the medication into the spacer and breathe it in when you are ready or in a number of short breaths rather than one large breath. People who have had to go to the doctor's surgery or hospital accident and emergency department with a severe asthma attack will probably be familiar with the **nebuliser** – a machine that pumps out a medicated mist that you breathe in through a mask. At one time the nebuliser was always used to treat severe asthma attacks, but many doctors now report that the latest designs of inhaler and spacer are as effective as the nebuliser. Nebulisers are still used to treat some elderly or very young people who cannot hold an inhaler.

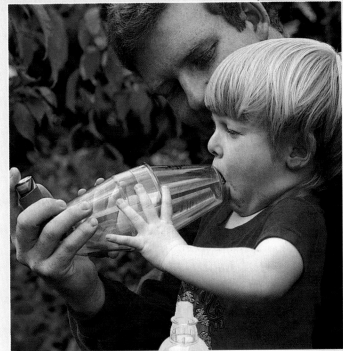

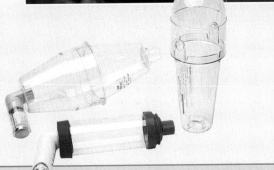

DIETARY SUPPLEMENTS

People with asthma should never stop taking prescribed drugs except on medical advice, but in some cases it may help to take vitamin C supplements as well. Some studies have suggested that a balanced diet with plenty of fruit and vegetables protects against asthma and some other lung diseases, and that eating more of certain types of foods and increasing consumption of vitamin C, magnesium and fish oils (Omega-3 fatty acids) can also improve symptoms.

LIVING WITH ASTHMA

The substances that trigger asthma attacks vary from one person to another. If you have asthma, you will be less vulnerable to an attack if you can identify your triggers and avoid them. There are many other ways in which you can make the condition easier to live with.
- Keep your home clear of dust and pollen. Avoid tobacco smoke.
- Avoid cats; their fur is highly allergenic.
- Managing stress and remaining calm helps to reduce the incidence of asthma attacks.
- Treat colds and flu promptly to reduce the chances of an attack.
- In winter, wear a scarf over your mouth and nose and breathe through the fabric to warm the cold air.
- Keep an asthma diary to help you to determine your asthma triggers and control your asthma.
- Regular exercise, especially swimming, is generally beneficial for asthmatics, but in some people exercise or exertion can trigger an attack.
- Some people with asthma find yoga and relaxation techniques beneficial in reducing asthma symptoms. A breathing method known as **Buteyko** is beneficial for some asthmatics.
SEE ALSO *Respiratory system*

CONTACT **Asthma UK** Providence House, Providence Place, London N1 0NT; helpline 0845 701 0203 9am–7pm Mon–Fri (www.asthma.org.uk)

Astigmatism

Astigmatism is an optical defect of the eye that causes sufferers to see objects distorted in size or leaning to one side. This usually occurs because the cornea of one or both eyes is unusually shaped.

Most astigmatism is present from early life; the degree of abnormality usually increases as the eye grows. The condition may also occur as a consequence of injury, certain diseases (especially those of the cornea) or ophthalmic surgery. A swelling in the lid such as a **chalazion** pressing upon the eye may cause astigmatism; in such cases, the astigmatism resolves once the lesion has been treated. Spectacles or contact lenses can effectively correct the symptoms of astigmatism in the majority of cases.
SEE ALSO *Eye and problems*

Asymptomatic

The term 'asymptomatic' is used to describe a disease process that produces no symptoms and therefore gives no sign that it exists. Many conditions are asymptomatic in their early stages. These include **diabetes**, high **blood pressure**, ischaemic heart disease (poor blood supply to the heart) and ovarian cancer.

Ataxia

Ataxia means loss of physical coordination. It may be caused by a developmental defect such as **cerebral palsy**. Another possible cause is injury to the cerebellum, the part of the brain that controls movement, or to the connections between that area and those that execute movements. An ataxic person retains the power to make normal movements, but is unable to control them. So, for example, an affected person might be able to grip an object firmly but be unable to manipulate it. **Dyspraxia** is a mild form of the condition, which is manifested as clumsiness or lack of coordination.
SEE ALSO *Brain and nervous system*

Atheroma

Atheroma is a condition in which deposits of **cholesterol** and blood cells develop on the artery walls. The walls then harden, making the arteries rigid – a process known as sclerosis – and the deposits enlarge into raised circular areas, called plaques. This eventually leads to a narrowing or blocking of the artery. If a crack

or fissure forms in a plaque, a blood clot may develop inside the artery. This is an arterial thrombosis, which may break away, leading to **coronary thrombosis** or **stroke**.

Atheroma affects most people by late middle-age, but causes no symptoms until it reaches the stage when the narrowing of an artery interferes with the circulation of the blood. Symptoms then depend on the part of the body affected. Complications such as heart attacks, strokes and circulatory problems can be delayed or prevented by adopting a healthier lifestyle.
SEE ALSO *Arteries and disorders*

Athetosis

Athetosis is the name given to involuntary slow writhing movements. These usually affect the hands and feet, but sometimes involve either one entire side of the body or all of it.

The movements are thought to be reflex actions – alternate grasping and avoidance moves. They occur as a result of damage to, or degeneration of, nerves in the brain that normally prevent them. Such movements tend to increase when the individuals affected are excited or under stress, and to diminish or disappear when they are relaxed or asleep. They may include:
- clenching and unclenching of the fists;
- facial grimaces;
- repeated swallowing;
- hand-wringing;
- writhing of the limbs.

The condition is usually associated with **cerebral palsy**, but drugs used to alleviate the symptoms of **Parkinson's disease** may bring some relief to sufferers.

Athlete's foot

Athlete's foot is a highly contagious **fungal infection** of the foot, which, despite its name, is not confined to athletes.

The infection is caused by a fungus known as *Tinea pedis*, which thrives in moist, warm areas of skin. It is easily spread wherever people walk barefoot – for example, in communal changing areas and showers, and in the bathroom at home. It can also be spread by sharing towels or shoes. More than 10 per cent of people in the UK are thought to be suffering from athlete's foot at any one time.
SYMPTOMS
The infection most often starts between the little toe and the one next to it, but it can spread around the foot and include the toenails.

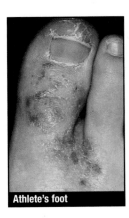

Athlete's foot

▲ **Itchy toes**
Athlete's foot, which usually begins between the toes, is the most common fungal infection of the skin.

It is characterized by:
- skin irritation and itching;
- red, raw patches of skin between the toes;
- an unpleasant smell;
- damp and soggy skin that may also crack, flake, bleed and become quite painful.

TREATMENT
The milder, most common form of athlete's foot can easily be treated at home.

What you can do
The important thing is to keep your feet clean: wash them carefully every day and dry them thoroughly after a bath or shower, especially between the toes. In addition:
- apply an over-the-counter antifungal cream, spray, liquid or powder to the affected area. Since the fungus burrows deep into the skin, make sure that you continue the treatment for at least ten days after all visible signs of infection have disappeared;
- wear cotton socks and change them every day, or more frequently if they become damp. Wear open-toed shoes whenever possible;
- never share towels or shoes; always wear flip-flops in communal changing areas or showers;
- clean and thoroughly rinse the bath or shower after use.

When to consult a doctor
Consult a doctor if the infection does not respond to self-help treatment or if it spreads to the nails and other parts of the body. The doctor may prescribe an antifungal cream or, if the infection has spread, an oral medication.

Complementary therapies
Tea tree oil has been shown to be effective in combating athlete's foot. Apply the oil neat to the affected area with a cotton bud, or soak the feet in a basin of water containing a few drops of the oil.

PREVENTION
Maintain good foot hygiene (see What you can do, above) and always wear flip-flops in communal changing rooms and showers.

COMPLICATIONS
If left untreated, athlete's foot can spread to other parts of the body, including the toenails, which turn yellowish brown and become brittle and difficult to cut. If the fungus spreads to the groin, it is known as 'jock itch'.

OUTLOOK
While treatment for athlete's food is usually effective, reinfection is common, and following preventive measures is recommended.

CONTACT **The Society of Chiropodists and Podiatrists** 1 Fellmonger's Path, Tower Bridge Road, London SE1 3LY (020) 7234 8620 (www.feetforlife.org)

Atrial fibrillation and flutter

Atrial fibrillation is a condition in which the conduction of electrical impulses through the upper chambers of the heart (the atria) is disordered and chaotic. This leads to an irregular contraction of the lower pumping chambers of the heart (the ventricles). In atrial flutter the atria contract very fast and regularly.

Both conditions reduce the heart's pumping efficiency. They become more common with age, affecting one person in 20 by the age of 75, and may be temporary, lifelong or intermittent.

SYMPTOMS
There may be no symptoms at all or the affected person may experience palpitations, faintness, breathlessness or chest pain.

CAUSES
Atrial fibrillation and flutter often have no obvious cause, and can be brought on by an infection or by excessive alcohol consumption. Disorders that may be the underlying cause include heart disease, respiratory disease, hypertension (high blood pressure) and thyrotoxicosis (see **Thyroid and disorders**).

TREATMENT
Consult a doctor if you have any concerns.

What a doctor may do
Tests, medications and procedures to diagnose and treat the problem may include:
- blood tests for heart or thyroid disease and for high blood cholesterol levels, which are a major risk factor for heart disease;
- a chest **X-ray**, electrocardiogram (**ECG**) or echocardiogram, which involves the use of **ultrasound** to examine the heart;
- drugs such as digoxin or amiodarone to slow down the heart rate or restore normal heart rhythm or **aspirin** or **anticoagulants** to reduce the risk of stroke;
- cardioversion – a short electric shock treatment, administered under anaesthetic, which may restore normal heart rhythm.

COMPLICATIONS
Atrial fibrillation or flutter may lead to low blood pressure or heart failure. It may also cause strokes from clot formation in the heart.
SEE ALSO *Arrhythmia; Heart and circulatory system*

Atrophy

Atrophy is a condition in which a limb, organ or tissue becomes shrunken and ceases to function as it should. It is caused by lack of stimulation – as is the case with muscles that waste away after damage to their nerve supply.
SEE ALSO *Muscular system*

Autism

Some autistic people are severely disabled, others have above-average intelligence, but all share problems of social interaction and communication, especially when it comes to recognizing and responding to others' emotions.

To varying degrees, autistic people fail to respond to their surroundings or interact with others. There may be hints of the condition from a very early age. A baby may fail to assume the usual anticipatory posture when about to be picked up, for example, and may arch away from its mother's grasp and avoid eye contact. Most symptoms of autism develop under the age of three. Affected children may be slow to speak, and speech may be impaired. Those severely affected do not develop speech and may appear not to understand what is said to them.

At around the age of four, non-autistic children develop the ability to empathize with others by mentally putting themselves in another's place. This social skill never develops in autistic people, although some may learn to understand others by deduction rather than by intuition. These kinds of non-spoken communication problems are known as 'Autistic Spectrum Disorders'. There are several other markers of childhood autism.
- Failure to indulge in 'pretend' play.
- Failure to join in communal games.
- Bizarre and obsessive interests, such as continuously rearranging or spinning objects.
- Preference for sameness – insisting on always taking the same route home or drinking from the same glass, for example.
- Greater interest in objects than people.
- Inability to deceive.
- Inability to understand metaphorical language, resulting in a literal interpretation of everything.

Autism is four times more likely to occur in boys than in girls.

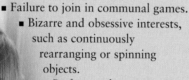

VARIOUS DEGREES OF AUTISM

People who are severely affected by autism may not be able to speak and may appear entirely unresponsive to their surroundings. Some spend almost all their time carrying out a single stereotypical movement such as rocking back and forth or twirling a strand of hair. Others can speak but use words in a very concrete way – for naming objects rather than expressing thoughts. Repetition of words or phrases spoken by another person is common.

Some may have average or above-average intelligence, and may be distinguished only by their social awkwardness; these people have what is known as high-functioning autism. Autism was thought to affect about five children in 10,000, although recent estimates suggest a much higher incidence. However, it is not clear whether these figures signify a sudden increase in the disorder or are simply due to the fact that autism is becoming more widely recognized.

Case study
Understanding an autistic child

An autistic child who does not understand the function of communication becomes frustrated.

Jon, an autistic 12-year-old, loved biscuits. The boy could not speak, so his father taught him to ask for a biscuit by pointing to the tin. Shortly after this, his parents were distressed when Jon's behaviour worsened – several times a day, they found him in the kitchen screaming with anger. Eventually his father discovered what was happening: passing the kitchen window he looked in and saw Jon pointing to the biscuit tin even though he was alone in the room. His father watched as the boy stood there for minute after minute, becoming agitated and then furious. Although Jon had learned that pointing brought him a biscuit, he did not realize that this was because his action communicated a message to another person who then acted on it. Jon had no conception of other people's 'inner worlds' – so, when pointing in the absence of another person failed to get him the goods, he could not understand why his desire was thwarted, and he became angry.

CAUSES

Autism is a neurodevelopmental disorder – that is, a condition caused by failure of normal brain growth rather than injury or other factors. There is a genetic component: if one child has autism, there is an increased likelihood of two to three per cent that a sibling will be affected. In boys, autistic symptoms may also be a feature of **Fragile X syndrome** – an inherited condition caused by a mutation on the X chromosome of either parent.

Women who contract infections such as rubella or cytomegalovirus during pregnancy have an increased likelihood of delivering an autistic child. The hereditary disorder tuberous sclerosis and the congenital disease **neurofibromatosis** have also been associated with autism, as have infantile conditions such as **febrile convulsions**.

Brain imaging and postmortem studies reveal subtle structural and functional abnormalities in the brains of autistic people, but the cause is not clear. One theory is that autism is caused by dysfunction in the frontal lobes of the brain, where data is combined in a way that makes it meaningful – for example, a house image is linked with its emotional associations to form the concept of 'home'. Autistic people are often unable to make such associations.

Some studies have suggested that the MMR vaccine may trigger the condition in some children, but the available evidence does not support this (see **Immunization**).

TREATMENT

There is no cure, but treatments such as special education, behaviour therapy and, in some cases, drugs can help to control some symptoms.

SEE ALSO *Asperger's syndrome; Brain and nervous system; Child development; Disability; Learning difficulties*

CONTACT **The National Autistic Society** 393 City Road, London EC1V 1NG; helpline 0845 070 4004 (www.nas.org.uk)

Autogenic training

Autogenic training is a form of meditation that can result in a state of deep mental and physical relaxation, found to be helpful in easing the symptoms of stress-related conditions such as anxiety, depression, irritable bowel syndrome, premenstrual syndrome and sleep difficulty. The technique has some similarities to self-hypnosis (see **Hypnotherapy**) but is easier to learn. It is usually taught by a qualified teacher to groups of about ten people over several weeks.

CONTACT **The British Autogenic Society** Royal London Homeopathic Hospital, Greenwell Street, London W1W 5BP (020) 7383 5108 (www.autogenic-therapy.org.uk)

Autoimmune disease

An autoimmune disease is any disease resulting from a fault in the body's **immune system** that causes the system to attack healthy body tissues.

Some autoimmune diseases seem to occur when cells become altered, perhaps as a result of a **viral infection**, so that the immune system no longer recognizes the cells as part of its own body. Women are generally more likely than men to be affected.

Symptoms and treatment of autoimmune conditions vary according to the particular disease. For example, in the case of rheumatoid arthritis, the joints become extremely painful, stiff and deformed. A wide range of treatments can be used, including anti-inflammatory drugs; the immune system can be suppressed with the use of **corticosteroids** or still more powerful immunosuppressant drugs.

Autonomic nervous system

The autonomic nervous system is part of the peripheral nervous system that controls the activity of internal organs and glands such as the heart, lungs and kidneys. Most of its effects occur without conscious thought from the higher centres of the brain, although some activities, such as anal and bladder control, have to be learned. Activities, such as heart and breathing rate, may also be controlled by overriding automatic mechanisms through **relaxation** and **meditation**.

The autonomic nervous system has two main parts – the sympathetic nervous system, which has stimulating effects, and the parasympathetic nervous system, which has relaxing effects.

SEE ALSO *Brain and nervous system*

Autopsy

An autopsy is the examination of a body after death. Its function is to establish the cause of death when this is unclear. An autopsy is also performed when death occurred violently or as a result of an accident.

An autopsy, or postmortem, is carried out by a pathologist, a doctor who specializes in the causes of disease and death. It is usually performed when there is doubt as to the cause of death, when it occurred suddenly or if there are any suspicious circumstances.

An autopsy is often distressing for the relatives of a deceased person. But there is a legal requirement to establish the cause of death, and the authorities have the right to insist that an autopsy be performed.

Many people feel more at ease when they fully understand the reasons why the procedure is taking place. An autopsy should cause no obvious disfigurement to the body.

THE LEGAL PROCEDURE

A death must be registered within five days at the register office in the district where it occurred. The registrar usually issues three certificates: one releasing the body for burial or cremation, one registering the death for social security purposes, and one that can be presented to banks, building societies and other organizations that might require proof of a person's death.

If there is any doubt about the cause of death, or in certain other circumstances, the registrar will not issue the certificates. Instead, the death will be referred to the coroner (a government official, usually a doctor or lawyer) who decides whether an autopsy is necessary. The coroner may also be informed of a death by a doctor or the police.

The coroner is informed if a death:
- was sudden, unnatural, unexplained or attended by suspicious circumstances;
- occurred during or following an operation or anaesthetic;
- was possibly due to an industrial accident, neglect or any kind of poisoning;
- happened while the person was in police or prison custody.

The coroner will also be contacted if:
- the deceased's GP had not seen the person within the last 14 days;
- the deceased was not treated by a doctor during the last illness.

THE ROLE OF THE CORONER

If the coroner is satisfied that the death was due to natural causes, and a doctor is able to certify this, the certificates will be issued immediately. If this is not the case, the coroner will request an autopsy. Relatives have no right to prevent an autopsy being performed, but they will be contacted by the coroner's office and told why it is being carried out.

The coroner is responsible for arranging the transport of the body from the place of death to the mortuary where the autopsy is carried out. The body should be stored in controlled conditions at all times.

THE AUTOPSY

The pathologist who carries out the autopsy will examine the body for evidence of the cause of death. Sometimes he or she will take a lead from the deceased person's doctor. For example, if the deceased was already known to be suffering from cardiac disease, only the heart might be examined. If there is no clear cause of death, the pathologist will perform a full autopsy, looking both for external signs, such as wounds or bruising, and internal ones, such as an undiagnosed cancer. Further tests may be carried out to check for the presence of substances such as drugs and alcohol which may have a bearing on the cause of death. Tissue specimens may be taken for microscopic inspection but no body parts should be withheld without the permission of the relatives. If the autopsy determines a natural cause of death, the coroner issues a certificate to the registrar. This enables the relatives to proceed with the funeral.

WHEN AN INQUEST IS HELD

If the autopsy shows that the death is not due to natural causes, the coroner is obliged by law to hold an inquest – a medical and legal enquiry to establish the facts surrounding the death. The coroner may adjourn the inquest and issue the necessary certificates for burial or cremation to allow the funeral to take place; in this case, the inquest will be reopened at a later date. Relatives may be called as witnesses to the inquest; it is obligatory to attend.

Autosuggestion

Autosuggestion is the practice of putting the mind into a relaxed and receptive state, then giving it a positive phrase or affirmation, such as 'I am getting better and better every day'. The aim of this is to stimulate the body's ability to heal itself. Some people have found it useful for reducing stress, breaking a harmful habit such as smoking, promoting better sleep or encouraging an optimistic attitude. You can be shown how to do this by a professional hypnotherapist (see **Hypnotherapy**) or a teacher of **meditation**.

SEE ALSO *Autogenic training*

Aversion therapy

Aversion therapy is a form of **behaviour therapy** that seeks to establish a connection in the mind of patients between their problem behaviour and an unpleasant response. For example, drugs that cause vomiting when they are mixed with alcohol have been used in aversion therapy to treat alcoholism. In theory, the intake of alcoholic drinks becomes associated with an unpleasant outcome in the mind of the alcoholic – and drinking declines. But the effectiveness of aversion therapy varies and it may change a person's behaviour for only a short period.

Ayurvedic medicine

Ayurvedic medicine has been practised for more than 2000 years on the Indian subcontinent, where it is still widely used. It is based on the idea that people can maintain good health through balancing physical, mental and spiritual energies in the body. This is done through lifestyle, diet and practices such as meditation and yoga. Ayurvedic practitioners believe that illness occurs when the body gets out of balance. Herbal medicine, massage with therapeutic oils, and purification techniques, such as fasting and enemas, may be used to help to restore the body's equilibrium and bring it back to health.

THE ORTHODOX VIEW

In the West, Ayurvedic practitioners are not usually medical doctors although they may have trained for three or four years. The system tends to be used for chronic conditions such as arthritis, general debilitation, certain women's health problems, asthma and irritable bowel syndrome. Ayurvedic medicine is not widely accepted and is not available on the NHS.

What's involved

Ayurvedic diagnosis is based on the practitioner's assessment of the natural balance of your energies. The practitioner will:
- question you closely about your lifestyle and diet, and take a full medical history;
- observe you, taking note of your posture and facial expression;
- check your pulses, tongue, skin, voice, abdomen, urine, stools and general appearance;
- recommend changes to your diet and lifestyle;
- carry out massage, purification techniques and other treatments.

CONTACT **Ayurvedic Medical Association UK** Eastern Clinic, 1079 Garratt Lane, London SW17 0LN (020) 8682 3876

▼ **Herbal healing** Ayurvedic remedies are often based on herbs and are sold ready-prepared or tailored to the individual.

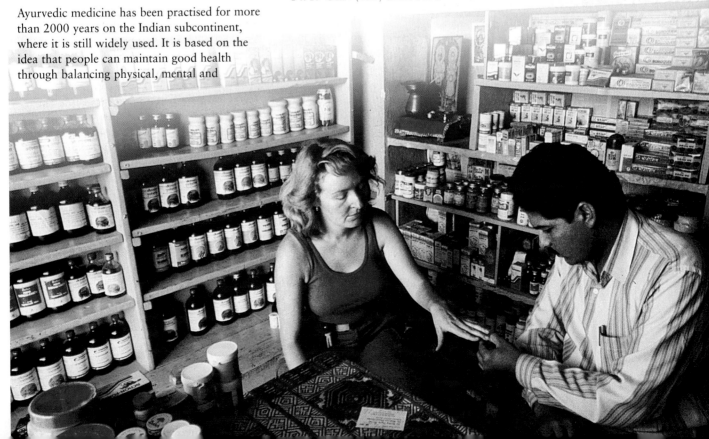

Babies and baby care

Caring for a newborn can be a challenging and even frightening experience, but the exciting developments in the first few months more than make up for the time and effort of early parenthood.

Adjusting to life with your baby is a gradual process that can make some parents feel inadequate at times, but you will gain confidence as your baby grows. In the first days and weeks after birth, regular home visits from a midwife and, later, a health visitor are a valuable source of support. More help and guidance can be found at the local child health clinic.

THE EARLY WEEKS
During the first few days after birth, babies are routinely tested for a metabolic disorder called phenylketonuria, which can cause brain damage if left untreated. The one-off test, which also looks for congenital hypothyroidism, involves taking a small amount of blood from the baby's heel. Some babies, including those who are particularly heavy or light, are tested for low blood sugar (hypoglycaemia), which can lead to fits. This test involves taking blood from the heel several times during the first 48 hours.

Several physical changes take place during the first weeks of life. For example, the cord shrivels up and, about ten days after birth, falls off. You will be advised how to keep the cord clean.

Most changes are perfectly normal but can be worrying – for example, blotches, spots or rashes may appear on the baby's skin, but these usually

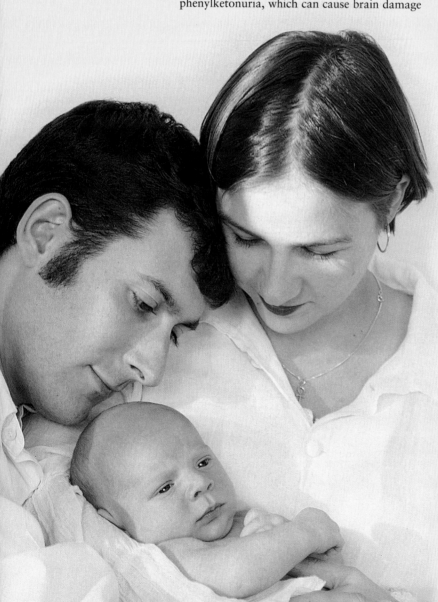

Self-help
Look after yourself

It is easy for the mother of a young baby to neglect her own needs, but it is important that she should take care of herself and get plenty of rest – particularly at a time when she is recovering from the emotional and physical upheavals of pregnancy and childbirth.

- Do only essential housework.

- Rest when your baby is sleeping.

- Encourage your partner to take time off work and involve him in the baby's care.

- Limit visitors. Put on your answerphone or hang a 'Do not disturb' notice on the door when resting.

- Accept any help that is offered – or, if necessary, ask for help.

- Don't neglect eating. Try to eat the kind of balanced diet you were advised about during pregnancy. Foods such as cereals, wholemeal sandwiches, cheese, yoghurts and fruit are nourishing and easy to prepare if you haven't the time or the appetite for cooked meals.

- Don't feel guilty about eating convenience meals or takeaways in the early days. Cook double quantities of food such as casseroles to freeze and eat later.

go away without treatment. Jaundice, resulting in yellowish coloured skin, normally clears up after about a week. Do not hesitate to consult your midwife, health visitor or doctor if you are concerned about anything.

CARING FOR A NEWBORN BABY

During the early weeks, it may seem that your baby does little more than feed, sleep, cry and wet or soil nappies. This period does not last long, and as you respond to your baby's needs you are helping him or her to feel safe and secure.

Some mothers do not fall in love with their babies instantly. If you feel nothing for your baby at first, don't panic or feel guilty. Just give it time. However, if you feel depressed or are worried that you might harm your baby, it is vital to talk to your midwife, health visitor or doctor. They will help you, not criticize you.

SLEEPING

Babies vary in the amount of time they sleep. On average, new babies may be awake for eight hours a day, and they usually sleep in stretches of three to five hours. If you put your baby to sleep in the cot while still awake, he or she will learn to fall asleep unaided. Babies who are used to being nursed to sleep may later refuse to settle easily.

Put your baby to sleep on his or her back. The move towards this rather than placing babies on their front has markedly reduced the incidence of cot death (**sudden infant death syndrome**).

CRYING

Babies tend to cry a lot in the early weeks of life because crying is the only way they can make their needs known. Gradually you will learn to distinguish between different cries – hunger, excessive heat or cold, a soiled nappy, loneliness, boredom, tiredness or overstimulation, and **colic**.

Factfile
Premature babies

Babies born before the 37th week of pregnancy are described as premature. They are categorized in one of three weight groups:

- 1500–2499g (3lb 5oz–5lb 8oz): low birthweight.
- 1000–1500g (2lb 4oz–3lb 5oz): very low birthweight.
- Below 1000g (2lb 4oz): extremely low birthweight.

Most premature babies are initially cared for in hospital. You may feel helpless, but the hospital staff will be keen for you to visit frequently and to touch, hold and feed your baby. You will be encouraged to breastfeed, if you can, or to feed the baby with expressed breast milk. Breast milk is better-tolerated than formula milk, reduces the risk of infection and contains a host of important factors not found in formula milk.

Before your baby is discharged from hospital, you will be expected to take responsibility for his or her routine care. Your baby's development will be assessed from the expected date of delivery rather than the actual birth date, but immunizations will be given, as usual, at 8, 12 and 16 weeks from the date of birth.

The most common reason for crying is hunger, which can be satisfied by a feed – but sometimes the baby cannot be pacified so easily. If the baby feels too hot or cold or is otherwise uncomfortable, being lifted up and comforted may be enough to restore equilibrium. When your baby is crying, follow your instinct and don't worry about 'spoiling' him or her if a cuddle is needed. Rhythmic movement or gentle massage may bring solace. Parents who respond quickly to their babies' cries have been shown to have babies who are more contented and secure.

If you feel your baby cries excessively or often appears to be in pain, seek medical advice. A baby with colic can be particularly hard to comfort, and it may be that you simply have to live with the problem, which usually resolves itself within a few weeks.

Fontanelle

The soft areas on the top of a baby's head where the scalp bones have not yet joined are known as fontanelles.

They may look vulnerable, but the 'soft spots' or fontanelles are covered by a very tough membrane, and they cannot be damaged during normal handling. It is usual for them to pulsate. The back fontanelle closes at six to eight weeks; the larger front fontanelle closes by 18–24 months.

Fontanelle

Feeding your baby

Feeds are times to relax with your baby and help you both to learn about each other.

Only breast milk or formula milk made from modified cow's milk should be fed to a baby under one year old. Ordinary cow's milk or other milks such as condensed or goat's milk do not contain the right proportion of nutrients. Soya-milk formula should be used only on the advice of a health professional. A new baby, whether breastfed or bottle-fed, can take about six weeks, sometimes more, to settle into a feeding pattern.

BREASTFEEDING

Breastfeeding brings many benefits to mothers and babies. Not all mothers find it easy, but with calmness and perseverance most challenges can be overcome. Midwives, health visitors and breastfeeding counsellors can give support.

Learning how to 'latch on'

A baby who is not properly attached, or latched on, to the mother's breast will chew or suck on the nipple, which can lead to soreness and other problems. New mothers often need time, patience and practice to get the baby to latch on correctly.
■ Before starting a feed, get into a comfortable position, such as sitting on an upright chair with your feet raised on a cushion. You may need extra pillows to support your back and arms, or to place across your lap for the baby to lie on.
■ If you had stitches after the birth, sitting on a pillow may be more comfortable. If you had a Caesarean, you may want to feed while lying on your side.
■ With the baby's body facing your body, and the baby's head and shoulders at the same level as your nipple, take the baby to your breast (not your breast to the baby) and gently prompt him or her to open the mouth. It may help to support your breast from underneath with your free hand.
■ A properly positioned baby will take in a mouthful of breast, including the nipple and much of the underside of the areola (the dark area surrounding the nipple). You will be able to hear the baby swallowing, and see his ears move.

Breastfeeding challenges

Problems with breastfeeding are not inevitable and can often be prevented by correct positioning and feeding on demand.

The most common challenge is sore nipples, but occasionally other problems such as engorgement (hardening of the breasts), a blocked milk duct or mastitis can arise (see **Breasts and disorders**). In these cases, ask your doctor or health visitor for advice. If breastfeeding is well established and you experience sore nipples or sharp shooting pains in the breast, check your nipples for **thrush**.

> It is normal for babies to lose some weight during the first few days of life. This is usually regained during the next ten days or so. Thereafter, the rate of gain is about 150g (5½oz) a week. In the average baby, birth weight roughly doubles by five to six months and trebles by the age of one year.

Expressing breast milk

You may need or wish to express breast milk if:
■ your baby is in a special care unit;
■ your breasts are engorged;
■ you are going out for several hours and want someone else to feed your baby;
■ you are returning to work and want to build up a regular store of milk.

Your milk can be expressed straight into a sterile bottle, a sterile plastic container or breast-milk freezer bags. The expressed milk can then be safely stored in a fridge for 24 hours or frozen for up to three months.

You can express milk by hand or with a hand pump, a battery pump or an electric pump. Expressing milk may be hard at first but it gets easier with practice. Before buying a pump, borrow or hire one to make sure that it suits you. To express by hand, support your breast with one hand and stroke downwards from the top of your breast towards the areola with the other hand; squeeze the lower part of your breast with your thumb and finger, pressing deeply to guide the milk out. Move your fingers and thumb progressively around the outside of your breasts.

Feeding facts

Breastfeeding, for just a few weeks or even days is worthwhile for your baby

How often should I breastfeed?
Feed on demand whenever your baby seems hungry, or feed (or express) when your breasts feel full. In the early days of a baby's life this may mean every two hours. Demand feeding also helps to prevent problems such as engorgement (hardness of the breasts).

How long should I feed for?
Don't limit or time feeds; if you do, your baby may not take in enough high-calorie hindmilk, which satisfies hunger and helps growth (as opposed to the watery foremilk, low in calories and fat, that gives a baby a drink at the start of a feed). Let your baby empty one breast completely before offering the other.

Can I build up my milk supply by offering formula?
On the contrary, the more you breastfeed the more milk your breasts make. If your baby seems hungry soon after feeding, check that he or she is latching on properly and feed more often.

BOTTLE-FEEDING FORMULA MILK

Follow the instructions on the packet and use the correct proportion of milk powder to water – otherwise the milk may be too weak or too concentrated. Bottles can be made up and kept in the fridge for 24 hours (discard unused feeds after 24 hours).

Test the temperature of the milk by shaking a couple of drops onto your wrist; it should feel just warm (not hot). Cuddle your baby and support his or her head and back with your arm as you gently insert the teat into the mouth.

After feeding, wash bottles and teats in warm soapy water and place them in a dishwasher – or, if your baby is less than six months old, sterilize them in a chemical solution or an electric steamer.

How much milk?

As a general guide, a baby needs about 150ml milk per kilogram body weight (2½ fl oz per 1lb body weight) per day. An easy way to calculate the correct amount in fluid ounces is to give about half your baby's body weight in pounds for each feed – for example, if your baby weighs 8lb, make up around 4fl oz of milk each feed. He or she will probably take more milk at some feeds and less at others. Never re-use leftover milk.

WEANING

Solid foods can be introduced gradually when your baby is between the ages of four and six months. By six months, a baby needs more iron and other nutrients than milk alone can provide. The aim at this stage is to introduce tastes and get the baby used to a spoon; first foods should

Feeding problems

Babies always swallow some air when they feed, and many bring up some milk with that air.

Wind If your baby suffers from wind, check that the teat hole in the bottle is not too large or too small. Make sure that the bottle is well tilted when feeding to stop air getting into the feed. Try not to let the baby wait too long for a feed: he or she may swallow air when crying. The best position for burping is over your shoulder – but protect your clothes with a rag.

Possetting Many babies bring back a small amount of milk after a feed; this is called possetting. If the baby is gaining weight, and the vomiting is non-forceful, don't worry. Possetting usually resolves itself once the baby is on solids.

Vomiting If your baby suffers from forceful or projectile vomiting, or appears to be in pain, contact your doctor.

be smooth and runny – baby rice or puréed fruit and vegetables, for example. Don't add sugar or salt to your baby's foods.

Once the baby is six months old, food should be mashed or minced – introducing soft lumps at this age encourages chewing and speech development and helps to avoid fussy eating later. If your baby is drinking less than 600ml (1 pint) of formula milk each day after the age of six months, or you are still breastfeeding, give five drops of combined vitamins A, D and C daily.

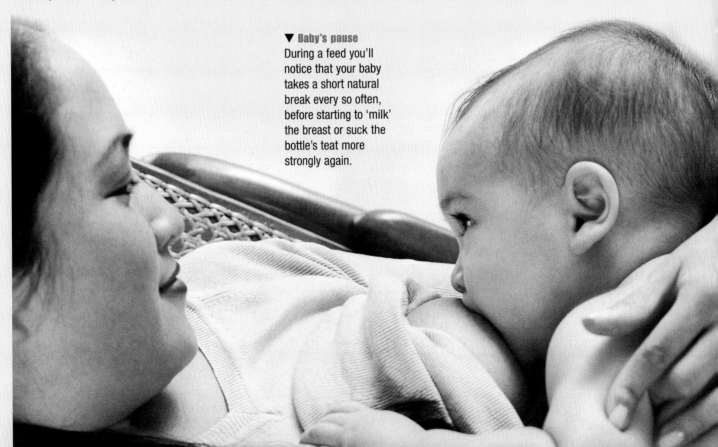

▼ **Baby's pause**
During a feed you'll notice that your baby takes a short natural break every so often, before starting to 'milk' the breast or suck the bottle's teat more strongly again.

Caring for your baby

Your baby relies on you to monitor and meet every daily need for warmth, comfort and security.

This small person, who has turned your world upside down, is, for now, completely helpless. But as you and your baby get to know each other, life will become easier and more predictable

BATHING

You don't need to bath your baby daily. Instead you can 'top and tail' – that is, clean the face, ears, the skin folds of the neck and armpits and nappy area, exposing only the parts you are washing. Always make sure that your baby's skin is quite dry before putting any clothes on. It is easier to dress a baby on a changing table or bed rather than across your knee.

NAPPIES

You can use cloth or disposable nappies, or both. Cloth nappies are cheaper and softer than disposables, and they can be used many times. Disposable nappies are convenient, with no laundering required, but they are expensive, occupy storage space, and are less friendly to the environment than cloth ones.

The number of stools passed varies and the appearance of a newborn baby's stools changes over a few days from meconium (the first dark green motions) to greenish brown, then yellow. There will probably be more than four stools a day, and two a day by four months. Breastfed babies may have twice as many stools as bottle-fed ones; these are often runny. If stools are hard or look like little pebbles, or none is passed for several days, consult your doctor or health visitor.

Nappy rash

This may appear as a red patch or as open spots, pimples or blisters. A nappy rash that will not heal may be infected with **thrush**, indicated by whitish spots or patches. To treat or help to prevent a rash, change nappies often, clean the area gently but thoroughly and apply a nappy-rash cream. Expose the baby's skin to the air frequently to aid healing. Avoid plastic pants.

How to bath a baby

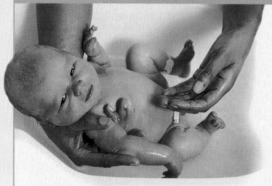

Many babies love bathtime: they relax and enjoy being washed in the soothing warm water.

1 Put hot and cold water in the bowl or bath, starting with cold water to avoid scalding. Check the water with the inside of your wrist or your elbow to make sure that it is comfortably warm but not hot.

2 Undress your baby except for the nappy and wrap him or her snugly in a towel, keeping the arms tucked away and leaving the head free.

3 Wash your baby's face with plain warm water and cotton wool. Wash the creases behind the baby's ears and around his or her neck.

4 To wash your baby's hair, tuck his or her body under your arm, supporting the back with your arm and the head with your hand. Hold the baby over the bath, wash and rinse the hair and pat dry.

5 Remove the nappy and clean the baby's bottom. Place your arm behind the baby's back, with your hand firmly holding the baby's arm that is further away from you. With your other hand supporting the legs and buttocks, lower the baby into the bath.

6 Keeping your arm around the head and shoulders, wash the baby's body; sit the baby up and, supporting the chest across your arm, wash the back.

7 Keeping one hand firmly on the baby's shoulder, slide the other hand under the buttocks and lift the baby out of the bath.

8 Dry your baby carefully, especially the skin folds. Rub oil or baby lotion into any dry areas of skin.

! Warning

Never leave young children alone in the bath – even for a moment. They can drown in two inches of water. If you have to go out of the bathroom, wrap your baby up and take him or her with you.

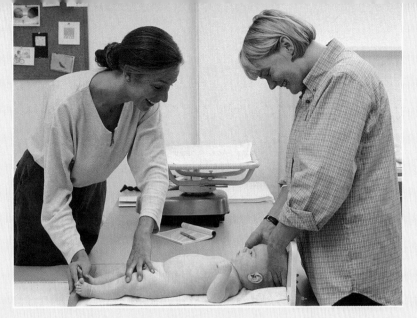

▲ Measuring growth
From the age of six to eight weeks onwards, your baby's length and weight will be measured by a doctor or health visitor during regular developmental checks at a GP surgery or health clinic. 'Centile' charts are used to record the measurements.

ILLNESSES
Most babies suffer brief and minor illnesses during the first year of life. If your baby has a fever or cold it is not usually necessary to consult a doctor. The following steps will bring relief:
- keep him or her cool (overheating can be dangerous);
- offer extra drinks of breast milk, diluted formula milk or water;
- give the recommended dose of paracetamol syrup for your child's age.

When to consult a doctor
If your baby is ill, you may need to call a doctor to your home urgently. But it is usually better to go to the surgery or to the accident and emergency department of your local hospital, where you are likely to be seen more quickly and the doctor will have more equipment to aid diagnosis. Consult a doctor urgently if your baby:
- has an unexplained rash;
- keeps crying and cannot be soothed, or has an unusual cry;
- has cold, clammy skin that is pale, grey or a dusky colour;
- has a temperature over 39°C (102.2°F) with rapid breathing or other signs of illness;
- passes blood or motions that look like redcurrant jelly;
- has severe diarrhoea and/or vomiting and is unable to keep fluids down;
- has a convulsion (fit) or seems floppy;
- has difficulty in breathing, is grunting, or turns blue;
- cannot be woken or is unusually drowsy;
- has a vacant or staring expression, or is unresponsive;
- has symptoms of **meningitis**. These include fever, vomiting and sensitivity to light.

Complementary therapies
Baby massage is an increasingly popular method of soothing and communicating with babies. Your health visitor can tell you about local classes.

Cranial osteopathy involves gentle manipulation and touch to identify and correct disorders within the body. It is mostly used to treat babies for feeding difficulties, colic, disturbed sleep and similar problems. But there is a lack of research evidence to support many of the claims made.

IMMUNIZATION
When children are immunized, they are given a vaccine containing some of the bacteria or viruses that cause a disease. These vaccines do not cause the disease itself but stimulate the body into producing **antibodies** against it.

During the first year of life, your child can be given vaccines to protect against diphtheria, tetanus, polio, whooping cough (pertussis), *Haemophilus influenzae* Type B (Hib) and meningitis C. Some children have adverse reactions to these injections, but serious complications are rare (see **Immunization**).

PHYSICAL AND SOCIAL DEVELOPMENT
In the first year, babies attain an astonishing number of developmental milestones, for example, babies learn to sit before, months later, they learn to walk. But children reach these stages at different times. Most babies are sitting by eight months of age, but some may sit as early as five months and others may not sit until ten months.

Many physical skills involving hand-eye coordination develop during the first year of life, enabling the baby to use hands and fingers for activities such as grasping and picking up. A baby can hear from birth and reacts differently to different sounds. At first, babies communicate only by crying, but they soon start making the little sounds that are the beginning of speech.

Social and emotional development is equally swift. Most babies return smiles and responses by the age of six to eight weeks and show likes and dislikes by 24–26 weeks. By their first birthday they can understand simple requests. Consult your doctor or health visitor if you are concerned about your baby's development at any stage.

SEE ALSO *Breastfeeding; Child care; Child development; Pregnancy and problems*

CONTACT **The Maternity Alliance**
Unit 3.3, 2–6 Northburgh Street, London EC1V 0AY; helpline (020) 7490 7638 (www.maternityalliance.org.uk)
The National Childbirth Trust
Alexandra House, Oldham Terrace, London W3 6NH; helpline 0870 444 8707; breastfeeding helpline 0870 444 8708 (www.nctpregnancyandbabycare.com)
La Leche League PO Box 29, West Bridgford, Nottingham NG2 7NP; helpline 0845 120 2918 (www.laleche.org.uk)

Bach flower remedies

Bach flower remedies are gentle, natural medicines that are thought by some to relieve challenging emotions – from rage or insecurity to self-absorption or disappointment. The process of choosing a remedy in itself helps people to recognize their emotions, which can be useful.

The remedies contain pure water, tiny traces of British plants or flowers – such as wild rose, elm, heather and holly – and brandy, which acts as a preservative. They can be added to water and sipped, or drops may be placed under the tongue. The remedies are available from most pharmacies and health food shops.

The range of remedies was developed in the 1930s by Edward Bach, a Harley Street doctor. Rescue Remedy – a ready-made mixture used for shock, fear or anxiety – is perhaps the best known; independent midwives often give it to women in labour. The remedies do not interfere with orthodox medical treatments or other complementary therapies. There are no reported side effects. But most orthodox medical opinion is sceptical about their effectiveness.

Flower power

Each flower remedy is thought to contain a subtle energy or life force and to heal by restoring inner harmony.

■ Physical disorder is seen as the outcome of an emotional or spiritual disorder. Practitioners use the remedies to promote spiritual equilibrium.

■ The remedies can be used to treat temporary emotional traumas such as bereavement as well as long-standing conditions.

■ There are 38 remedies in all, and they can be used singly or in combinations of up to five.

WHAT'S INVOLVED

Many aromatherapists, homeopaths and herbalists are trained in the use of Bach remedies.
■ Consultations last up to an hour. You may need only one visit or a course of treatments.
■ A therapist will ask you about your life, your medical history and how you react to particular situations, and will then recommend a remedy or mixture of remedies on the basis of your personality and how you are feeling.
SEE ALSO *Aromatherapy; Herbalism; Homeopathy*

CONTACT **The Dr Edward Bach Centre**
Mount Vernon, Sotwell, Wallingford, Oxon
OX10 0PZ (01491) 834678
(www.bachcentre.com)

Back and back pain

The back is a well designed structure vulnerable to modern living and back pain is an ever-present fact of life for many people.

The spine is a column of bones that extends from the skull to the pelvis, forming, in profile, a shallow S-shape. It has several functions. It supports the head and allows the body to remain upright, and it provides anchorage points for the ribs, the ligaments and the muscles of the back. This allows very flexible movement of the trunk – forwards, backwards, down to the side and back up, and in a circular movement. The spine also protects the spinal cord (see **Brain and nervous system**) and stores red **bone marrow** to form red blood cells and minerals.

VERTEBRAE AND DISCS

The spine contains 33 bones, or vertebrae. With the exception of the atlas and axis (which are uppermost and act as pivots for the head), all the vertebrae are similar, although they become larger as the spine runs down the body to cope with the increasing weight. Each has five main parts:
■ the body or centrum, the main cylinder-shaped part of the vertebra;
■ the vertebral arch, the space through which the spinal cord passes as it runs down the back from the brain;
■ two transverse 'processes', bony projections from the body that provide points of contact for ligaments and muscle tendons;

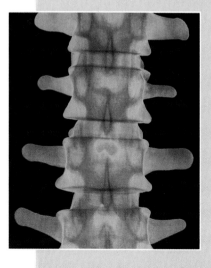

◀ **Vertebral structure**
Each vertebra consists of a short weight-bearing cylindrical core called the body or centrum. This has bony projections, or processes, to which the muscles and ligaments are attached. Separating the vertebrae are discs encased in cartilage.

Main support

The central structure of the back is the spine. It is held together by joints and ligaments and supported by both large and small muscles.

The cervical spine consists of seven vertebrae, which support the head and neck. The uppermost two are the atlas and axis, which form pivots for the head

The thoracic spine serves as attachment points for the ribs and comprises 12 vertebrae

Lumbar spine has five vertebrae that form the lower back

The sacrum has five fused vertebrae, forming a strong joint for the pelvis

Coccyx or tailbone is formed from four vertebrae

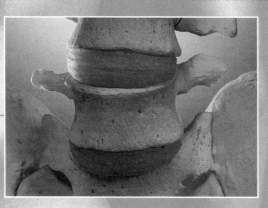

▲ **Vulnerable spot**
Pain often occurs in the lower lumbar region and the sacrum, which links the spine to the pelvic bone.

■ one spinous process, which can be felt at the back of the spine.

Discs sit between the vertebrae. The discs have a soft, jelly-like centre that is 95 per cent water, and an outer casing made of tough but flexible elastic **cartilage**. They mould themselves into the available space (rather like a balloon full of water) to allow for movement of the spine, and also to act as shock absorbers.

The vertebrae are also linked by facet joints. These bind each set of transverse processes with the ones above and below. Spaces between the vertebrae near the facet joints allow the nerves to enter and leave the spinal cord.

CAUSES OF BACK PAIN

Back pain is often the result of lifestyle, ageing or an accident. It can also be caused by conditions that directly affect the spine, including **ankylosing spondylitis, Paget's disease, cancer** and what is popularly known as a slipped disc (see **Prolapse**). In cases of prolapse, it is not in fact the disc that is displaced but the jelly-like centre, which is forced by pressure through a defect in the disc's outer ring and squashed backwards to press on a spinal nerve.

Other conditions may cause pain in the spine even though the spine is not directly affected. These include **influenza**, heart problems, lung problems, kidney problems, an inflamed pancreas or gall bladder, and gynaecological problems. A fractured vertebra or a slipped vertebra (where one vertebra slips out of its position in the spinal column) may be caused by an accident or a fall.

Lifestyle factors

A sedentary lifestyle puts extra pressure on the lumbar spine, especially if you tend to slouch rather than sitting up straight. Pressure in intervertebral discs increases by 50 per cent when you sit with a straight back compared to when you are standing. But when you slouch forward it increases by 150 per cent. Over time, the extra pressure damages the vertebral joints, especially the facet joints, and causes muscular tension, spasms and pain.

People who take excessive exercise or who do a lot of exercise without building up their fitness gradually may suffer soft-tissue damage in their backs. This is because their muscles are not strong enough to cope with the extra demands placed upon them. The muscles may tear or go into spasm, pushing the surfaces of adjacent facet joints down onto each other. The affected joints become inflamed and painful.

Looking after young children involves a lot of bending, lifting and stretching, which can lead to

Types of back pain

Back problems can have many causes and usually give pain and a degree of immobility. The different types of back pain can be felt in specific places or over wider areas but it is usually possible to establish the nature of the problem from the type of pain and whether it is short or long term.

- **A sharp, localized pain** that changes with movement is likely to be caused by dysfunction of a facet joint. The pain eases if a movement takes pressure off the joint and worsens and spreads if the pressure is increased.

- **Chronic back pain** can come and go or it can be felt continuously. It can vary from a dull, muscular ache to a sharp twinge when certain movements are made. Poor posture, weak or imbalanced muscles, soft-tissue damage from unaccustomed exercise, and degenerative conditions such as osteoporosis and osteoarthritis are all possible contributory factors.

- **General soft-tissue damage** to muscle fibres, tendons and ligaments produces localized acute pain and stiffness that subsides over a few days.

- **Immobility and severe pain,** and what some sufferers have described as the feeling that the back could 'snap in half', can occur when the back locks in one position. The cause is a dislocation at the facet joints of a vertebra, most often as a result of a sudden movement that involves bending and twisting at the same time.

- **Muscle spasm** can cause painful hot spots, sometimes called 'trigger points', in the back muscles. These are tender areas that are painful to the touch and can restrict movement. This type of pain occurs after an injury, when the muscle fibres go into spasm to prevent any further damage being done.

- **General stiffness** in the back, especially first thing in the morning, is often the result of osteoarthritis in people aged over 50, or of ankylosing spondylitis in younger people. But it can also be the consequence of unaccustomed exercise the previous day.

- **Pain combined with pins and needles**, numbness and muscle weakness can be the result of nerve damage caused by pressure on a nerve or the spinal cord, when it is known as a central spinal stenosis. The pain can also run down the back of the leg and under the foot.

- **An acute, sharp, burning pain** that is relentless and often immobilizing and debilitating; is usually caused by inflammation of a spinal nerve or pressure on it where it leaves the vertebra.

About 1.1 million people in the UK are registered as disabled as a result of back problems – more than for any other cause.

back problems if care is not taken. Fashion can also take its toll – wearing high heels increases the pressure on the lower spine. Menstruation can trigger back pain, and a woman's altered posture in later **pregnancy** can result in back pain and **sciatica**.

Osteoarthritis

Osteoarthritis is a common diagnosis of back pain. It is sometimes called spondylosis when it occurs in the spine. As a result of wear and tear, cartilage in the discs and facet joints starts to harden and turn into bone, and bony spurs grow out from the facet joints. These restrict movement and sometimes even impinge on a nerve. (See **Arthritis**.)

Osteoarthritis is to some extent a natural part of ageing; most people aged over 50 have the condition to some degree, even if they have no symptoms. The condition can develop at any point in the spine, but the lumbar and cervical vertebrae are the most vulnerable to ageing. Other causes include a previous injury, a condition such as ankylosing spondylitis, overuse and poor posture.

Osteoporosis

Osteoporosis is a condition in which the calcium content of bones is reduced, making them thinner, less dense and more likely to fracture. When the vertebrae lose density, they start to crumble, distorting the spinal curves and causing muscle spasms. As the process continues, the vertebrae impact and may trap the spinal nerves, causing considerable pain as well as immobility. (See also **Spine and disorders.**)

TREATMENT FOR BACK PAIN

If you have chronic back pain, the general advice is to carry on as best you can with your normal life, but to avoid lifting and carrying. According to the Royal College of Physicians' Faculty of Occupational Medicine, the majority of back pain sufferers do not need bed rest. Contact your doctor if the pain worsens or persists for longer than 48 hours.

If you experience acute, severe back pain or symptoms of sciatica (see Types of back pain, page 144), rest in bed if you can do nothing else. If the pain remains after 24 hours, seek medical advice.

What you can do

■ Lay a hot water bottle on the affected area, or use a heat lamp.

■ Take over-the-counter medications, such as codeine, paracetamol or ibuprofen – a painkiller and anti-inflammatory – to relieve pain from injury and help the muscles to relax. Or use embrocation creams, which can be rubbed into the skin to relieve stiffness. Hot or cold sprays can be used for the same purpose.

■ Arrange for a **massage** to ease muscle tension and spasm.

■ Consider using a back brace or belt. These will restrict the small muscle movements and help the muscles to relax. A corset can be used as a temporary measure only, because long-term use will further weaken the spine's muscular support, making it more vulnerable to stresses.

■ Do graduated exercises to strengthen your back and stomach muscles (see Strengthening your back, page 146).

■ Use relaxation techniques – long-term back pain may be related to stress and other psychological problems, such as **depression**.

When to consult a doctor

■ Get someone to call an ambulance immediately if you suspect that you have hurt your neck or back following an accident or fall. Do not move. Wait for emergency assistance.

■ Go to casualty if your car has been hit from behind while you were sitting in it, even if you feel unhurt – you may have a whiplash injury.

■ Call your doctor if a sudden, immobilizing pain has not improved after 24 hours of bed rest.

■ Call your doctor if a continuous pain has not improved after 48 hours of home treatment.

■ See your doctor if you suspect you may have osteoporosis, you are postmenopausal or have a family history of osteoporosis or have an existing spinal problem.

What a doctor may do

■ Give you a general physical examination, looking particularly at the strength of your muscles and your range of movement.

■ Arrange a bone density scan to rule out osteoporosis.

■ Suggest you wear a corset as a short-term measure – these are available on the NHS.

■ Inject a **corticosteroid** drug into any painful trigger point.

■ Prescribe **drugs** such as: anti-inflammatories, muscle relaxants, **tranquillizers**, strong **painkillers**, **steroids** or **antidepressants**, as appropriate.

■ Refer you to a physiotherapist, a muscularskeletal physician or to a surgeon or neurologist.

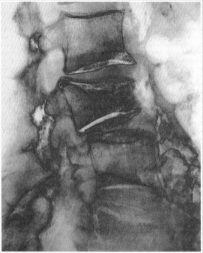

▲ **Spinal distortion**
A lumbar vertebra in the spine of a 65-year-old woman has become compressed and wedge-shaped as a result of osteoporosis.

Physiotherapy

The most common treatment for back pain is **physiotherapy**. Physical methods are either used alone or in conjunction with painkillers. Treatment can include manipulation, exercises, **ultrasound** and **hydrotherapy**. Physiotherapists also give training on good posture, teach correct lifting techniques and give advice on how to protect your back while performing everyday activities in the home and garden, while travelling and in the office.

Complementary therapies

Increasingly, complementary techniques are being used to treat back pain. These include **osteopathy**, therapeutic **massage, chiropractic, acupuncture** and the **Alexander technique**. Osteopaths, for example, work on the assumption that many back problems are caused by the displacement of one vertebra in relation to another, and that they can be relieved by identifying the site of the dislocation and applying pressure to reduce it.

Surgery and alternatives

Surgery is used only as a last resort for back problems. There are a variety of options.

■ An injection of a corticosteroid drug and a painkiller into the facet joint to relieve inflammation. This is administered under a local anaesthetic by an anaesthetist.

■ An injection of chymopapain, a chemical derived from the pawpaw fruit, into a prolapsed disc to digest its soft centre. The success rate is 80 per cent, and removes the need for surgery. But the disc remains thin and vulnerable to damage.

These simple daily exercises can help strengthen the muscles supporting the spine and reduce the risk of back problems. Do not strain or force the movement, though: stop if you feel discomfort.

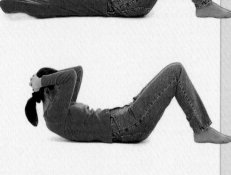
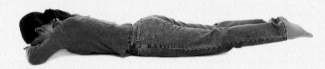
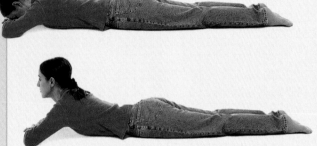

2 Turn over onto your back and bend your knees at right angles, with your feet on the floor. Place your hands behind your head and lift your head, shoulders and shoulder blades up off the floor – for safety, do not attempt to sit right up – then lower them slowly and carefully. Repeat five times.

1 Lie on your stomach on the floor with your hands laced under your forehead. Slowly raise your head and shoulders about 20cm (8in) – no more – off the floor, then lower them slowly back to the floor. Repeat five times.

3 With your head on your hands, raise both legs about 15cm (6in) off the floor, then lower slowly. Repeat five times.

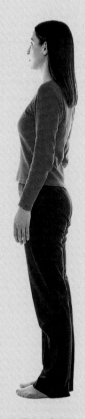

▲ **Natural grace**
If you strive to maintain the correct standing posture at all times, it will eventually become instinctive.

■ An emergency operation called a discectomy to remove a prolapsed disc. This will free a trapped nerve when there is a risk of neurological problems affecting other parts of the body.
■ An operation called a spinal fusion to fuse together two or more vertebrae. This can be done using a bone graft from the hip bone or with pins and screws. It will stabilize a slipped vertebra or stop an unnatural spinal curve becoming worse.
■ An operation called a facetectomy to remove bony spurs around a facet joint caused by osteoarthritis. This allows more room for the spinal cord or nerves.

PREVENTING BACK PAIN
In many cases, back problems can be prevented by adopting good posture, using the correct techniques when lifting heavy objects, exercising for strength and flexibility, and taking certain practical measures during everyday life.
The importance of good posture
Bad posture is the most common cause of chronic back pain – and potentially the easiest to avoid.

The back has four natural curves that give it the ability to absorb the stresses of maintaining an upright posture. The sacral and thoracic vertebrae curve backwards (outwards when seen from the side) – they are called primary curves because they are present at birth. The cervical and lumbar vertebrae curve forwards (inwards when seen from the side) and develop shortly after birth as a baby learns to lift the head and sit.

If the back is held either too straight or in an exaggeratedly curved position, the spinal column and its muscles and ligaments are unable to absorb the everyday shocks and stresses of gravity, walking, sitting and weight-bearing, and so become distorted. When the shoulders and upper back become rounded, the unnatural curve is known as a **kyphosis**; the excessive inward curve of a 'hollow back' is called a lumbar lordosis; a sideways curve to the spine is called a scoliosis.

Over time, the muscles and ligaments become either too long or too short and the bones and joints become liable to excessive wear and tear. The result is damage to tissue and bone – leading to back pain.

Poor posture quickly becomes a habit, and starts to feel correct even when it is not. Many people find that they need to relearn good postural habits, perhaps with the help of a physiotherapist or an Alexander technique teacher. But you can train yourself to adopt and maintain good posture.
Sitting and standing tall Try to avoid slumping in a chair, hunching over a desk or table, or walking around with hunched shoulders. Imagine there is an invisible cord from the top of your head to the ceiling lifting you into a tall, relaxed posture.

Use a full-length mirror to check that the various parts of your body are properly aligned. Start by standing up straight with your feet hip-width apart and pointing forward.
■ The knees should be pointing forwards, but should not be locked back.

Whether you are lifting a small child or a box of heavy books, always try to use the correct technique to protect your back.

1 Check the weight of the object before you lift it. Stand in front of the object, as close to it as possible, with your feet in a wide stance on either side of it. Place one foot further forwards than the other to improve your balance.

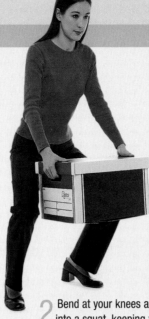

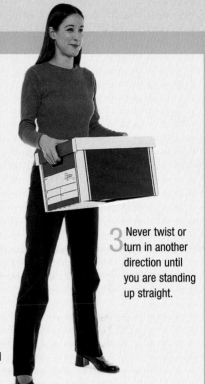

2 Bend at your knees and hips into a squat, keeping your back straight. Grip the object securely and use your leg muscles to stand up straight while bringing the object in towards your body.

3 Never twist or turn in another direction until you are standing up straight.

■ The shoulders should be level, back and down but not forced back.

■ The back should be straight when viewed from behind but should retain its natural curves when viewed from the side.

■ The crown of the head should be the highest point with the chin neither tucked in nor stuck out. Eyes and ears should be level, and the neck held straight and long.

■ The abdominal and buttock muscles should be tucked in to support and brace the spine and to prevent an exaggerated curve in the lower spine.

Lifting technique

Incorrect posture while lifting causes more acute back problems than any other activity. The reason for this is that lifting exacerbates any existing weakness in the back, such as muscular weakness or imbalance, a ligament strain, or damage caused by wear and tear. But a combination of lifting and certain other activities can cause damage when there is not necessarily a weakness. Manual workers are most at risk of developing chronic back pain because they are often required to lift a variety of heavy objects using different techniques. (See Correct lifting techniques, above.)

Regular exercise

The abdominal and back muscles brace the spinal column and allow it to absorb the stresses of movement. In order to function correctly, both abdominal and back muscles must be of equal strength and carry an equal degree of tension so that one set can relax and lengthen while the

other shortens and tightens. Any weakness or imbalance puts strain on the ligaments and joints. Taking regular exercise therefore plays an important part in maintaining a healthy back. (See also Strengthening your back, page 146.)

Day-to-day care of your back

Follow these simple rules to minimize the chances of developing problems with your back.

■ Check your posture frequently.

■ Avoid holding any one position for too long.

■ Avoid standing still for long periods – sit or put one foot up on a stool or raised object to reduce the pressure on your back.

■ Ensure that while you are at work any chair that you use regularly protects your back: your feet should touch the ground; the back rest should support your spine; and the chair should be deep enough to support your thighs.

■ If you use a computer, make sure that the screen is at the correct height: you should not have to look down at it.

■ Before embarking on gardening or household chores, warm up with some stretching exercises.

■ Use long-handled tools to take some of the strain out of gardening.

■ Stay fit and keep within the weight limits for your height and age to reduce spinal stress.

CONTACT **BackCare** 16 Elmtree Road, Teddington, Middlesex TW11 8ST (020) 8977 5474 (www.backcare.org.uk)

Bacterial infections

Many diseases are caused by bacteria, which are single-cell organisms too small to be seen by the naked eye. Most are harmless to people and some are beneficial, but others, abundant in the air, soil and water, cause disease by releasing substances harmful to human cells.

SYMPTOMS

Bacterial infections can cause:
- skin problems, including rashes;
- breathing problems;
- high temperature or fever;
- stomach pains;
- headaches;
- genito-urinary problems.

COMPLICATIONS

Many bacterial infections can cause further damage to the body and its organs – including **whooping cough, meningitis, botulism, tuberculosis, typhoid fever, Legionnaire's disease** and **syphilis**.

OUTLOOK

Early treatment with **antibiotics** is often essential for bacterial infections, which may otherwise cause permanent health problems.

SEE ALSO *Immune system and disorders*

Avoiding the spread of infection

Bacterial contamination most commonly occurs through physical contact – from unwashed hands to dirty kitchen utensils.

The simplest, most everyday actions can spread infection.

- Touching or shaking hands with another person.

- Contaminated food infecting the digestive tract.

- Touching food with dirty hands – this will also allow bacteria from the intestine to spread.

- Inhaling droplets breathed, coughed or sneezed out by an infected person – **diphtheria** and **whooping cough** are caught through the lungs in this way.

- Sexual contact. Micro-organisms that enter the genito-urinary system include those causing **sexually transmitted diseases** such as syphilis, pelvic inflammatory disease and gonorrhoea.

- Through hair follicles, cuts and deep wounds.

To prevent infection, you should take the following steps.

- Wash your hands thoroughly and often.

- Store vegetables and meat separately and prepare them on separate chopping boards.

- Cook meat until it is well done.

- Use a handkerchief if coughing or sneezing.

- Wash wounds with **antiseptic**.

- Get yourself immunized against bacterial diseases such as **tetanus**.

Bad breath

Bad breath, also known as **halitosis**, is unpleasant mouth odour, often caused by poor oral hygiene, sinus problems or, occasionally, stomach problems. If you think that you suffer from bad breath, you should talk to a dentist. If the cause is related to inattentive dental care, you may be advised to see a hygienist.

SEE ALSO *Dentist and dentistry*

Balance

Balance problems may be experienced as toppling or stumbling or, more subtly, by a feeling of unsteadiness, nausea or dizziness. Keeping one's balance depends on a continuous, complex process that involves the eyes, ears, brain and nerves.

Information about body position is fed to the brain in a continuous stream from the eyes, movement sensors in the inner ear, and nerves in the skin, joints and muscles. From this, the brain computes what the body must do to stay 'on course', and transmits instructions back to the limbs. The process involves several areas of the brain, including the cerebellum and the sensory and motor cortices.

ONSET AND DURATION

A balance problem may occur suddenly or over a number of years. Problems with balance are very common in old age, and slow-developing imbalance in later life is unlikely to signify anything sinister – it affects the majority of people over the age of 85. However, any sudden loss of balance should be treated as a medical emergency unless there is an obvious cause such as intoxication. If imbalance develops over several weeks, a doctor should be consulted.

CAUSES

Because it involves so many different parts of the body, the balance system may be disrupted by a very wide range of conditions. It is associated with many different illnesses and can be one of the first signs that a person is tired, intoxicated or very stressed.

Ear disorders

- **Ménière's disease**, an abnormal increase in the pressure in the inner ear.
- **Labyrinthitis**, inner ear inflammation.
- **Otitis media**, inflammation of the middle ear.
- **Blocked ears**, which may be caused by a buildup of wax.

Nerve disorders

- Inflammation of the nerve fibres, which may be due to viral or bacterial infection.
- Nerve degeneration, which may signify vitamin B deficiency.

■ **Multiple sclerosis**, which causes damage to myelin nerve sheaths.

Blood and circulation disorders

■ **Anaemia**, which reduces brain oxygen levels.

■ Blood poisoning, caused by infections or environmental toxins (see **Septicaemia**).

■ Cardiovascular disease, which reduces blood flow to the brain.

■ **Hypoglycaemia**, or low blood sugar.

■ High or low **blood pressure**.

Brain abnormalities

■ A **stroke** that affects the brain's sensory or movement areas.

■ A tumour that affects the sensory or movement areas.

■ **Motor neurone disease**, which causes death of the brain cells required for movement.

TREATMENT

Treatment will vary, depending on the underlying condition.

SEE ALSO *Blood and disorders; Brain and nervous system; Heart and circulatory system; Ear and problems*

Balanitis

Balanitis is a condition in which both the head of the penis (glans) and the foreskin become inflamed. It can affect men of all ages, and in boys occurs most commonly around the age of three or four years. Unusual among circumcised males (see **Circumcision**), balanitis is best avoided by keeping the penis clean, especially under the foreskin.

Balanitis can develop from infection following damage to the skin surface caused by:

■ poor genital hygiene;

■ a tight foreskin (**phimosis**);

■ skin disorders such as **Reiter's disease**;

■ an allergic reaction to a particular soap or washing powder or to the latex or spermicides in condoms;

■ sexual activity – although the condition itself is not transmitted sexually, the **candida** fungus can be transmitted and cause localized inflammation.

Most cases clear up without treatment – although you should abstain from sex until the skin has healed. If after a week or two you are still feeling discomfort or are worried that the irritation could be caused by a **sexually transmitted disease**, see a GP or visit your local genito-urinary medicine (GUM) clinic.

Antibiotics, **antifungals** or **steroids** may be prescribed.

SEE ALSO *Fungal infections; Penis and disorders; Reproductive system*

Baldness

Baldness, also known as androgenic or male pattern baldness, is a common condition that usually poses no health problems. As many as 25 per cent of men in the UK are noticeably balding by the age of 30, and 65 per cent by the age of 60. Baldness can, more rarely, affect women.

SYMPTOMS

In men, the hairline recedes from the front or, less often, from the top of the head; in women, hair tends to thin out all over.

CAUSES

There is a strong hereditary element in baldness, with the biggest influence generally on the mother's side. The trigger, most frequently, is hormonal. Although the mechanism is unclear, **testosterone**, which increases body hair and reduces scalp hair, is involved.

Other causes can include:

■ serious illnesses, infections or fevers;

■ **chemotherapy** and **radiotherapy**;

■ stress;

■ excessive shampooing or blowdrying.

TREATMENT

There is no cure but treatments include:

■ hair grafts (the relocation of hairy skin to bald patches), sometimes in tandem with scalp reduction (the removal of bald skin);

■ artificial hair fibre implants;

■ wigs – an effective, short-term solution to, for example, hair loss caused by chemotherapy;

■ Minoxidil, which is rubbed on the scalp. This is the only male baldness drug licensed in the UK for sale without a prescription. Research suggests that, after four months' use, it stopped hair loss in about 70 per cent of users and stimulated some growth in half the people who tried it;

■ early tests of dutasteride, a drug which interferes with the enzymes that cause hair to thin dramatically in later life, look promising.

Anyone considering drug treatments for baldness should research the latest available products thoroughly with a sympathetic GP or trichologist, a hair specialist.

COMPLICATIONS

■ Side effects can arise from any drug treatment.

■ **Depression** is a relatively common response to baldness, especially in young men, women and children.

CONTACT **www.malehealth.co.uk** This website includes an introduction to drug treatments.
The Institute of Trichologists Fraser House, Netherall Road, Doncaster DN1 2PH
08706 070602 (www.trichologists.org.uk)

Hair care

You cannot prevent receding hair but you can slow down the process.

■ Treat remaining hair gently, especially when it is wet.

■ Comb rather than brush your hair.

■ To keep hair healthy, ensure your diet contains sufficient protein and iron (see **Diet**).

■ Wearing your hair short is usually better than trying to disguise a bald patch.

Bandaging

Bandaging is used to control bleeding, keep dressings in position, apply pressure, provide support or prevent movement. Bandages can be used in several ways:

- as a triangular cloth to make a sling;
- as a broad wrapping to cover a large area, for example, to bind a fractured leg to the other leg as a temporary splint;
- as a narrow strip, for example, when wrapped around a limb to hold a dressing in place;
- as padding, for example, around an embedded piece of glass in a wound.

CHANGING DRESSINGS

Severe wounds or skin infections are usually treated in hospital or by a visiting nurse. When changing the dressings covering a wound, it is important to avoid the risk of infection. Always do the following.

1 Wash your hands thoroughly, preferably using an antiseptic skin cleanser.
2 Place within reach the dressings (sterile dressings should be contained within unbroken packaging until you are ready to use them), antiseptic cleanser, cotton wool and clean bandaging, as required.
3 Ensure that the area to be dressed is accessible and the person is comfortable.
4 Carefully remove the existing dressings and dispose of them immediately.
5 Gently clean the area as necessary with antiseptic cleanser.
6 Place the dressing over the wound with the sterile side down, and secure with a bandage or adhesive tape.

BANDAGING A WOUNDED LIMB

1 Wind one end of the bandage around the limb once, leaving a short end dangling; this will keep the dressing in place and hold the bandage in position.
2 Holding the dangling end clear, wind the other end of the bandage around several more

---

Warning

Check for signs that a bandage may be tied too tightly.

- Fingernails or toenails have blue colouring.
- Fingers or toes appear pale.
- The end of a bandaged limb feels abnormally cold.
- The person complains of tingling or numbness.
- The person cannot move his or her fingers or toes.

---

times until the dressing is comfortably secured and the two ends of the bandage are next to each other.
3 Tie the two ends of bandage together.

Bandages often need to be applied firmly to provide some pressure, but if they are tied too tightly they can stop blood circulation to a limb, which can be dangerous. Look out for signs of restricted blood supply (see Warning, below left), checking every ten minutes or so for the first few hours after bandaging. If there is any indication of impaired blood supply, loosen the bandage and re-apply with a little less tension in the winding.

SEE ALSO *FIRST AID*

Barber's rash

Known also as folliculitis, barber's rash is an infection of a man's beard area. A similar but usually less serious condition is called razor bumps. Both barber's rash and razor bumps can make shaving difficult and painful.

Barber's rash is caused by infection of the hair follicles by a common skin bacterium, *Staphylococcus aureus*. Infection, and re-infection, often occur through using razors or towels previously used by an infected person.

Razor bumps are caused when facial hair curls and grows back into the skin to cause inflammation. This condition is particularly problematic for men with curly hair.

SYMPTOMS

- In barber's rash, there is itchiness, redness, swelling, multiple small pus-filled blisters and occasionally boils. The condition usually starts on the upper lip, but can spread across the face. It can also occur on the groin and thighs.
- Razor bumps are characterized by redness and inflammation and sometimes by infection.

TREATMENT

- Always use clean towels and razors.
- Wash your face twice daily with hot water and antibacterial soap.
- If you have razor bumps, always shave 'with the grain'. Do not pull your skin taut to get a closer shave.
- Shave less frequently or use an electric razor if it is more comfortable.
- Growing a beard usually solves the problem.
- If your skin is infected and these self-help methods fail to cure the condition, seek medical advice. Your doctor may prescribe an antibiotic cream, a course of antibiotic tablets, or both treatments .

COMPLICATIONS

Scarring can very occasionally result from untreated barber's rash.

Barbiturates

Barbiturates are powerful **central nervous system** depressants – that is, they depress (reduce) central nervous system activity. They were once used extensively as sleeping pills, general anaesthetics, sedatives in the treatment of **anxiety**, and as **anticonvulsants** for epilepsy.

Today, they are rarely prescribed because of their dangers: in overdose they can be lethal, and they can rapidly cause psychological and physical dependence. **Benzodiazepine** drugs are often used instead.

ADVICE ON USAGE

If you are taking barbiturates, be aware that:
- they interact with a variety of drugs, and high doses taken with alcohol can cause fatal coma;
- use of barbiturates when pregnant can harm the baby;
- stopping barbiturate treatment or treating barbiturate addiction involves a gradual reduction in dose as withdrawal symptoms can be severe.

DRUG ABUSE

When taken orally or injected into veins, barbiturates produce symptoms similar to drunkenness. Some people take barbiturates (known as 'barbs' or 'downers') recreationally. Because of the risk of abuse and the dangers of overdose, they are on the controlled **drugs** list.

SEE ALSO *Addictions*

Barium investigations

A barium investigation is a diagnostic test used to investigate disorders of the stomach, gullet or bowel. There are three types of barium investigation:
- the barium swallow (used when a doctor wishes to examine the gullet);
- the barium meal (for investigating the stomach and upper intestine);
- the barium enema (used to examine the rectum and lower intestine).

WHAT'S INVOLVED

The first and second types involve drinking a thick, white, often mint-flavoured solution; in the third the solution is pumped into the rectum. The liquid (a solution of barium sulphate) shows up on **X-rays**: abnormalities of the digestive tract can be seen on X-ray pictures or viewed on an imaging device called a fluoroscope.

For meals and swallows, people are asked to drink up to two cupfuls of the solution and may also be given an injection to paralyse the gut temporarily. The part of the digestive system to be investigated must be empty; for a barium

enema, a laxative may first be given to empty the bowel. X-ray pictures will be taken immediately or within 45 minutes depending on where in the gastro-intestinal tract the investigation is centred. Barium investigations cause no discomfort at the time, but patients may find that they have constipation for a day or two afterwards.

Barium meals are not performed as commonly as they once were. Increasingly, medics are using a fibre-optic device called a gastroscope instead. It examines the oesophagus and stomach for any suspected growths and can take tissue samples at the same time.

Since bacteria are the most common cause of stomach **ulcers**, and since barium meals and gastroscopes do not detect bacteria, doctors generally do not use these invasive techniques when first investigating possible stomach ulcer symptoms.

SEE ALSO *Digestive system; Oesophagus and disorders; Stomach and disorders*

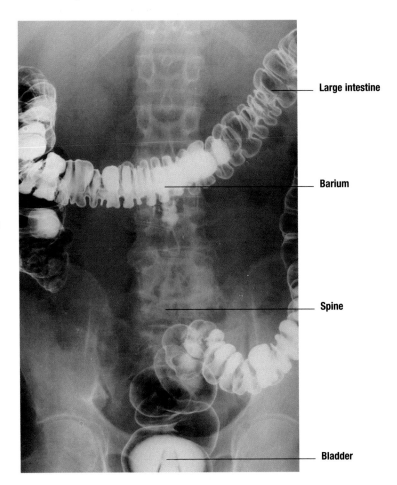

Large intestine

Barium

Spine

Bladder

▲ **Diagnostic meal**
This X-ray image shows part of the large intestine highlighted after a person has taken a barium meal. Medics can use the image to diagnose a digestive complaint.

Barrier creams

Barrier creams can be used to protect the skin against irritants, chapping, haemorrhoids (piles), bedsores, toxic substances, nappy rash and pressure sores. Some creams contain added **antiseptics** to prevent or counter infection.

Barrier creams such as Sudocrem and Vasogen are widely available without a prescription. They commonly have a petroleum-jelly base and often include substances that repel water, such as silicone compounds. Sometimes lanolin is added to these preparations – some people are allergic to it and may therefore experience a degree of irritation.

Bartholin's cyst and abscess

A Bartholin's cyst is a swelling, usually on one side only, of the external female genitals (vulva). The swelling begins as a painless **cyst** but may become infected and enlarged, resulting in a very painful **abscess** that may interfere with sexual intercourse. It is caused by a blockage in one of the Bartholin lubricating glands, which are positioned at the back of the vulva. It is most common in women of reproductive age.

Any swelling in this area that does not go away after a few days should be medically examined. You may be prescribed a course of **antibiotics** to treat the condition or referred to a consultant gynaecologist, who will consider surgical removal of the cyst or abscess. To obtain relief at home, try sitting on a cold compress or in a lukewarm bath.

Basal metabolic rate

The basal metabolic rate (BMR) is the rate at which an individual expends energy while at rest in order for essential activities such as brain function, breathing, digestion and heartbeat to take place. BMR is influenced by age, gender (men have a higher BMR than women), weight, stress and hormones. It determines his or her tendency to lay down fat stores in the body, and is a balance between the efficient use of calories from food and expenditure of stored energy reserves.

Basal metabolic rate is controlled by the hormone thyroxine, sometimes known as the metabolic hormone, which is essential for the normal functioning of the body. A deficiency of thyroxine can cause **myxoedema**, a slowly developing disease that leads to lack of energy and a thickening of the skin.

SEE ALSO *Thyroid and disorders*

Bates method

The Bates method is a series of eye exercises designed by American ophthalmologist William Bates in the early 20th century. It may be recommended by practitioners of **homeopathy**, **naturopathy** and the **Alexander technique**.

Patients are taught to relax their eyes by covering them, when closed, with the palms of the hands. There are exercises involving controlled blinking and movements of the eyes or of the whole head.

Some Bates method exercises might help with minor eye problems such as 'tired eyes' after long periods in front of a computer terminal. But most doctors believe that more effective solutions to that problem would be to ensure that you take regular rest breaks and have good lighting at your work station.

SEE ALSO *Eye and problems*

Bazin's disease

Bazin's disease (erythema induratum) is a rare form of **tuberculosis**, which does not affect the lungs. In the UK there are around 20 cases of Bazin's disease each year.

The classic symptoms are deep red, bruise-like swellings, usually on the shins. Sufferers may also feel generally unwell, but although infected they are not infectious.

A doctor will arrange a **biopsy** to confirm the condition. Treatment consists of a course of **antibiotics**, which may take six to eight months to complete. If the treatment is continued correctly, most cases are cured.

BCG vaccine

The BCG vaccine is administered to provide immunity from **tuberculosis**. Its full name is Bacillus Calmette-Guérin vaccine. The vaccine is produced from live but weakened cattle tuberculosis bacteria, which do not cause the disease in human beings but stimulate the production of specific **antibodies**. These antibodies react with the human tuberculosis bacteria to give the recipient of the vaccine natural resistance to the disease.

The BCG vaccine is used (following a skin test) for routine vaccination of children, usually between the ages of 10 and 14, and for other people at risk. It is given by injection, generally into the upper arm. Within two to six weeks, a small swelling appears, which heals after six to twelve weeks to leave a small scar.

SEE ALSO *Immunization*

Bedbugs

Bedbugs are wingless insects with flattened, oval-shaped bodies measuring about 5mm (¼in) in length. Bedbugs bite human beings and other mammals to feed on their blood. The bugs hide in soft walls, bedding, mattresses and furniture by day, and come out at night, when most blood feeding occurs. The bugs are a pale brown colour and become red brown after consuming blood. Their bites look like little red bumps and can sometimes occur in a line on the body. They usually cause itchiness, but bedbugs are not known to transmit disease.

Bedbugs are generally associated with substandard housing and poor hygiene. Walls, bedding and other infested areas are often marked with black and brown spots of excreta and excess blood. To deal with an infestation of bedbugs, call a qualified pest control officer, who will apply an insecticide.

Bedsores

Bedsores are, initially, areas of skin irritation that develop on immobile people confined to bed. They are also known as pressure sores or decubitus ulcers. People at risk include those with a serious debilitating illness, people who have been paralysed (for example, following a stroke or spinal injury) or those in a coma.

Bedsores result when pressure from the body interferes with the circulation of blood to areas of flesh over bony prominences such as the heels, the base of the spine, the shoulder tips or the elbows. The sores start off as redness on the skin, but these marks become purple before breaking down and ulcerating. Turning the person over at least once every two hours and using rippled bed mattresses, cushions, pillows and sheepskin padding help to prevent bedsores. Treatment may involve the use of **antibiotics**, **ulcer** dressings and surgery to remove dead tissue and apply skin grafts.

SEE ALSO *Skin and disorders*

Bedwetting

Bedwetting (nocturnal enuresis) is defined by doctors as the involuntary wetting of the bed at night by a child over the age of five years. It is a common problem that can cause considerable distress to both children and their families.

Most children master daytime bladder control between the ages of two and three. Staying dry throughout the night can take longer: up to the age of five bedwetting is considered normal.

Before children can stay dry during the night they have to recognize and respond to a full bladder while asleep. This is done either by 'holding on' until morning or by waking up and urinating. Most children who wet the bed grow out of it as they get older.

CAUSES

The reason why some children wet the bed is not fully understood, but factors may include:
- genes – bedwetting runs in families;
- sleep disorders;
- anxiety or psychological problems;
- a deficiency of a hormone called vasopressin, which reduces secretion of urine when present in the body in normal amounts;
- developmental immaturity;
- diabetes or a urinary tract infection.

TREATMENT

Although treatment is not normally given before the age of five years, there are a number of general measures that parents and children can take to cope with bedwetting.
- Ask your doctor to test your child's urine to exclude any disease.
- Be reassuring, involve the child in the treatment and give praise for dry nights.
- Do not restrict your child's fluid intake: the bladder tends to adjust to receiving less fluid and therefore holds less. The Enuresis Resource and Information Centre recommends that children drink around six or seven cups of fluid each day so that their bladders learn to hold a larger capacity. Fizzy drinks and those containing caffeine should be avoided at night because these can act as diuretics and stimulate the kidneys to produce more urine.
- Try fully wakening your child at a slightly different time each night – this may reduce the number of wet beds.

A doctor or school nurse may suggest other things you can do. For example:
- star charts – your child is awarded a star on a chart every time he or she stays dry at night;
- an alarm to wake the child up when urination begins. Alarms can be effective but may take up to 16 weeks to work. For developmental reasons they are recommended by doctors only for children over the age of seven years;
- medicine, either tablets or a nasal spray, can reduce the amount of urine passed.

SEE ALSO *Child care; Child development; Urinary system*

CONTACT **Education and Resources for Improving Childhood Continence (ERIC)** 34 Old School House, Britannia Road, Kingswood, Bristol BS15 8DB (0117) 960 3060 (www.eric.org.uk) The centre offers information and advice and sells a selection of alarms.

Factfile
Bedwetting

Wetting the bed is very common in childhood.

- One in seven 7-year-olds regularly wets the bed.
- One in eleven 9-year-olds regularly wets the bed.
- Between one in 50 and one in 100 fifteen-year-olds and older regularly wets the bed.
- Children have a 40 per cent chance of bedwetting if one parent wet the bed as a child and a 70 per cent chance if both parents did.
- Bedwetting affects almost as many boys as girls, depending on the age group.

Behaviour problems in adults

Abnormal or problem behaviour is hard to define – who is to say when people are behaving abnormally and when they are merely being eccentric? But when their behaviour begins to constitute a danger to themselves or to others, then medical steps can and should be taken.

It can be distressing when a friend or relative begins to act strangely, especially if the behaviour is violent. The person may have aggressive outbursts or threaten self-violence, while remaining oblivious to the fact that this behaviour is upsetting others.

Behaviour problems are not always of a violent nature, however, and may include essentially passive changes such as the decline in activity that often accompanies **depression**. Previously busy and sociable individuals may lose interest in work, hobbies and relationships, begin to neglect their appearance, personal hygiene or diet, and become generally apathetic. Such people may seem unable to recognize familiar places or people, become confused and disoriented and suddenly unable to cope with ordinary tasks such as shopping or cooking. This behaviour may be accompanied by prolonged misery, persistent anxiety, general irritability or episodes of extreme, bubbly cheerfulness followed by correspondingly deep periods of unhappiness.

Other types of problem behaviour involve opting out of normal social constraints and rules. Some people seem to lose their inhibitions, hugging strangers or wandering around with no clothes on. They may plunge into self-destructive or risk-taking habits, often abandoning work or family duties – for example, becoming

▼ **Constant handwashing**
Unusual behaviour such as repetitive hand-washing or extreme anxiety when routine is disrupted may be the outward expression of an underlying disorder.

Older people with behaviour problems

A range of problems can affect older people's behaviour, including loss of short-term memory, depression, confusion and delirium.

Behaviour problems in older people may be caused by an emotional trauma such as bereavement or a major life change such as moving house, by the onset of a progressive illness such as dementia, by the drugs they are taking and interactions between them, or by prolonged hospitalization.

Dementia is often assumed to be the cause of behaviour or emotional problems in older people – but there are a number of treatable conditions with very similar symptoms that can be mistaken for dementia. These include depression, brain tumours, subdural haematoma (a swelling caused by blood pooling in the membranes of the brain) and vitamin B deficiency. A thorough assessment by a specialist in older people's mental health, a psychogeriatrician, may be necessary to check that a problem has not been misdiagnosed as dementia.

heavily reliant on alcohol or drugs, embarking on gambling or spending sprees that run up huge debts or taking up dangerous sports without proper preparation.

Many of these types of behaviour are accompanied by mental disturbance – people see things that aren't real, hear voices, develop irrational beliefs, become paranoid or lose themselves in grandiose plans that have little hope of fulfilment. Some develop obsessional or compulsive habits such as checking and double-checking that the gas is turned off, or the doors are locked.

ASSESSING PROBLEM BEHAVIOUR
Some of the behaviours described above, such as losing minor social inhibitions, may be harmless – and even charming – in some circumstances. As a general rule, unusual behaviour becomes a problem when it poses a threat of harm to others; brings the individual into conflict with the law; has a detrimental effect on the person's work,

study, health or relationships. It is also a problem when the person's behaviour is causing distress and difficulties for family, friends, neighbours or colleagues.

CAUSES OF BEHAVIOUR PROBLEMS

Sometimes unusual behaviour has a physical cause. Quite commonly the behaviour can be a reaction to prescribed drugs – if a friend or relative begins to act oddly, try to find out if he or she has recently begun taking new medication.

Illness such as **delirium** or an injury such as a blow to the head can also cause changes in an individual's behaviour. Other possible physical causes include **poisoning and gassing,** for example exposure to **carbon monoxide,** or accumulation of toxins such as mercury or lead in the blood.

Abuse of alcohol or recreational drugs is another possible cause – people may act unpredictably under their influence, and regular abuse can have physical effects associated with problem behaviour, for example, nutritional deficiencies in alcoholics can be a cause of behavioural changes. This can also affect people suffering from **eating disorders.**

Troubling and challenging behaviour can also be a sign of mental health problems such as depression, **phobia** or **anxiety** or of mental illness such as **dementia** or **schizophrenia.**

HOW TO SEEK HELP

People with behavioural problems may well be unwilling to accept that they have a problem, and you may need to seek help on their behalf. The family GP may be able to help. If the individual affected can be persuaded to cooperate, the GP can perform a range of tests to establish the cause of the problem and arrange treatment. This may involve medication, referral to a counsellor, psychiatrist or psychologist or voluntary treatment at a mental hospital. Behaviour therapy can sometimes help – art, music or drama therapy can channel anger or negative emotions accompanying depression, and promote self-expression. If the behaviour proves to have a physical cause, **homeopathy** can help. Consult a qualified homeopath. Changes in diet or use of **vitamin dietary supplements** can correct a dietary deficiency or imbalance. It is advisable for family members and others affected by the behaviour problem to seek help and support for themselves.

If the people whose behaviour is causing distress have a treatable mental disorder and represent a danger to themselves or others, they may be treated compulsorily (without consent) under the provisions of the Mental Health Act. A GP or an approved local authority social worker can arrange for a **mental health** assessment to see whether such an action is appropriate.

Case study
An unexpected side effect

Paula thought her brother's scruffy appearance and listless behaviour were signs of depression, but his behaviour had a hidden cause.

Mark was 45 with a high-flying job in an international telecommunications company. He seemed to thrive on the pressure and frequent travelling – although after a checkup Mark's doctor prescribed medication to control his blood pressure. When Mark was made redundant, his friends feared the worst. But he appeared to adapt very well. He took a marketing job at a local charity, started evening classes in Spanish cooking, and picked up the gardening he had loved as a boy.

However, one day when his sister Paula visited she found him sitting in semi-darkness. The house was cold and Mark had obviously been living on little more than toast and biscuits. His garden was becoming overrun with weeds and he appeared to be neglecting himself, too – his clothes were stained and he hadn't shaved for several days.

Paula was worried that her brother had become depressed, especially as he seemed listless and rather confused. Eventually she persuaded him to see his GP, who remembered that Mark had recently been given some new blood pressure tablets and guessed that the tablets had caused an adverse reaction that affected Mark's mood. The medication was changed and within days he was his normal cheerful self again – back at work at the charity, busily setting about ridding his flowerbeds of weeds and cooking Paula a celebratory paella.

SEE ALSO *Alcohol and abuse; Anorexia nervosa; Behaviour problems in children; Behaviour therapy; Cognitive behaviour therapy; Counselling; Dementia; Diabetes; Diet; Drugs, medicinal; Eating disorders; Head and injuries; Obsessions and compulsions; Paranoia; Psychiatric disorders; Psychoanalysis; Psychology; Psychological therapies*

CONTACT **Carers UK** Ruth Pitter House, 20–25 Glasshouse Yard, London EC1A 4JT; Carers line 0808 808 7777 10am–12pm and 2pm–4pm Wed & Thurs (www.carersonline.org.uk)
Mind 15–19 Broadway, London E15 4BQ; Mind*infoline* 0845 766 0163 9.15am–5.15pm Mon–Fri (www.mind.org.uk)
Rethink 28 Castle Street, Kingston-upon-Thames, Surrey KT1 1SS; National Advice Line 0845 456 0455 (www.rethink.org)

Behaviour problems in children

All children have a capacity for mischief, and naughtiness is a perfectly normal way of exploring the limits of acceptable conduct. Such behaviour constitutes a problem only when there is a danger of social or physical damage to a child or others.

Problem behaviour is difficult to define, because what is acceptable in one family may be regarded as outrageous in another. But children are generally reasonable people, and will aim to obey whatever rules parents lay down. Think what might be the cause if a child shows a worrying pattern of behaviour, or if it is getting worse. For example, if a child is persistently aggressive towards a sibling, could it be due to jealousy, boredom, tensions in the family that the child is picking up on, or unrealistic expectations on the part of the parents?

TEMPER TANTRUMS

Most children have uncontrollable fits of anger from time to time, but some are more prone than others to outbursts of kicking, screaming or throwing things. Temper tantrums are usually a passing phase, which begins at about 18 months and can last a year or so. Many parents feel that frustration lies at the root of the 'terrible twos'. Young children have real desires that they cannot quite express, and they are subject to rules and injunctions that they are not equipped to understand. They cannot see, for example, why they can empty a box of toys onto the floor but are not allowed to empty a bag of groceries.

Hard as it may be, ignoring tantrums is a good way of dealing with them. A child is more likely to give up on throwing tantrums if it proves to be an ineffective strategy, so don't use bribes or give in. Staying calm and avoiding making threats or smacking the child will mean less stress all round. Once the tantrum is over, make sure that your child knows you still love him or her, but that you dislike the behaviour.

Preventing tantrums

If your child has frequent tantrums, avoid trigger situations. For example, don't press your child to share a treasured toy. Also, decide when it is important to be firm: insist that a child holds your hand in the street, for example, but don't worry about odd socks if your child really wants to wear them.

Unclear rules from adults can be an underlying cause of tantrums, so both parents should try to act consistently. A child may find it confusing if, say, the mother buys sweets at the supermarket but the father won't. Going for too long without food may trigger tantrums so take a snack and drink when you go out with your child. Tantrums may also occur if there are too many activities in the day or a child misses a nap; don't expect too much of your child and allow time for a rest.

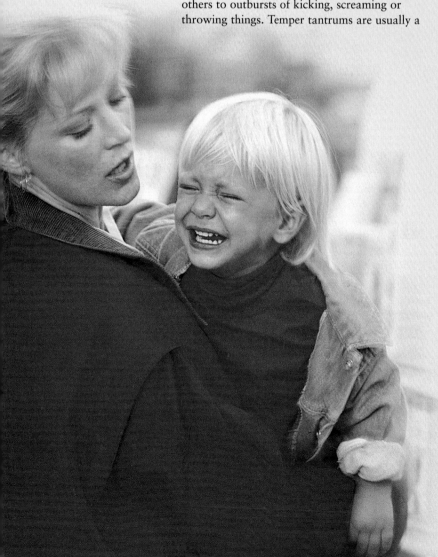

◄ Infant rage
Temper tantrums in public places can be a nightmare for parents, but do stay calm. You may feel embarrassed, but most people will sympathize rather than judge you or your child.

BREATH-HOLDING EPISODES

Some children hold their breath when they are crying, feeling upset or in a temper. When this occurs, the child's face turns red, then changes to white or blue. These spells may begin in babies as young as 6 months, peaking between 12 and 18 months, and can continue until the child is 3–3½ years old. In some cases, the child becomes stiff or floppy, and may pass out for a few seconds before starting to breathe again. These episodes are frightening for parents but will not normally harm the child. Discuss the behaviour with your doctor: as long as your doctor is sure that there is no underlying medical cause of the breathlessness and other symptoms, ignore a child who is having a breath-holding spell. If your child passes out, keep a close watch but move away when he or she starts to regain consciousness.

AGGRESSION

Violent behaviour can be due to something as simple as undeveloped social skills. For example, children aged under two years do not understand the concept of sharing and may become aggressive if they see another child playing with their toys. But a toddler who has started showing signs of aggression needs to know that this behaviour is unacceptable.

■ If you see your child about to bite or kick, issue a sharp and unequivocal 'no'.

■ Take your child into another room and talk about the behaviour. Even if he or she seems not to understand, the message will sink in over time.

■ Consider whether there is a reason for the behaviour, such as a new baby in the family. You may need to make a special effort to prevent older children from feeling neglected when a young baby is demanding much of your attention.

■ If children are fighting over toys, distract them with another.

■ Take pre-emptive action – for example, put away favourite toys when other children visit.

HEADBANGING AND HEAD-ROLLING

It is not unusual for children aged 6–18 months to bang or roll their head in a rhythmical way before going to sleep or if they are tired. Headbanging is alarming for parents, but the habit is harmless and usually resolves itself by the age of four.

Some children bang their heads to attract attention when they are upset. But most have the sense not to bang their heads so hard that they hurt themselves. If necessary, pad the sides of a child's cot, or put padding against a wall. If your child starts to bang the side of the head, check that he or she is not suffering from an ear infection that is causing pain.

Consult a doctor if your child's habit worries you, or if it continues after the age of four.

Encouraging good behaviour

Parents can help to foster good behaviour in their children with consistent and thoughtful reactions to everyday family issues.

Do

✓ Give your child firm boundaries so that it is clear what you will and will not tolerate.

✓ Be consistent, and if you make a threat carry it out. Parents need to agree on boundaries and sanctions.

✓ Give reasons why you have forbidden something. 'Because I say so' isn't good enough.

✓ Think before you say 'no', then stick to it.

✓ Praise positive behaviour, however infrequent, to raise self-esteem.

✓ Give children their own responsibilities to make them feel special – it could be walking the dog.

✓ Try to spend individual time with each of your children with no interruptions.

✓ Be realistic about children's academic abilities and concentrate on things they are good at.

✓ Allow your children to bring friends home so that you know who they are spending time with.

Don't

✗ Bribe your child to behave well.

✗ Physically punish your child. Banning television or withdrawing other privileges is more effective.

✗ Apply too much pressure by organizing too many out-of-school activities – children should have time to relax and daydream.

✗ Criticize your child in front of other people.

✗ Try to choose your child's friends.

✗ Give attention only for challenging behaviour.

JEALOUSY

Many older siblings feel left out when a new baby comes along. It is hard for a first child of any age to let go of exclusive relationships with its parents. But jealousy becomes a problem only if it manifests itself in disruptive reactions such as hitting a new baby, reverting to infantile behaviour or becoming physically destructive.

Try to anticipate jealousy. For instance, move a child out of your bedroom to make way for a new baby before, not after, the baby is born. Think about the cause. Do you always pick up the younger child first? Do you frequently compare one sibling with another, or take one's side against another? Children pick up on any hint that a parent's love or attention is being distributed unequally.

The pre-teen years

The pre-teen years are the time when a child's horizons expand beyond the home and the securities of family life.

Behaviour problems can appear suddenly and unexpectedly, and it can come as a shock to parents if a previously well-behaved child becomes aggressive, refuses to go to school or starts to lie or steal. Such behaviour is often a response to some unexpressed unhappiness or anxiety, so any strategy for dealing with problem behaviour must look for these causes as well as deal with their manifestations.

STEALING

If your child is stealing, you need to act quickly. A child who steals from school could end up damaging his or her educational career, and stealing from shops may land an older child in trouble with the police.

Talk to your child to find out the reason for stealing. Some children steal in order to gain the attention that comes with being caught, but the cause is not always psychological: stealing may be done as a silly dare or to gain favour with friends. Bullying can also be at the root of it: bullies sometimes force their victims to steal.

If your child is caught shoplifting, you should insist that he or she goes back to the shop with you to return the item, or that the child pay for it and apologizes to the shopkeeper. Most children will find this experience so mortifying that they will be disinclined to steal again.

Persistent stealing, particularly in children old enough to understand the moral fault involved, usually has some deeper cause. It may need investigation with the help of a psychotherapist, who will help the child to explore the issues behind their behaviour.

LYING

Fantasizing is a normal, and harmless, part of a child's development, but deliberate lying should be discouraged. Children of six or seven inhabit a different moral universe from adults. They believe that the more implausible the lie, the more reprehensible it is – so it is worse to say that you have seen a flying elephant than to claim you did not eat the chocolate in the fridge. Parents should gently make clear the difference between things that are not true because they are stories, and things that are not true because they are deceit.

By the age of seven or eight, children understand that telling lies can have real and unpleasant consequences for other people. But they may still tell lies because they are afraid that they will get into trouble or lose face, or that people won't like them if they tell the truth. They generally have a clear intuition that this kind of deception is wrong. Parents can do much by example: displaying a disapproving attitude to dishonesty to underline their child's almost innate sense of right and wrong.

REFUSING TO GO TO SCHOOL

Going to school can be an ordeal for some children and they may refuse to go or pretend to be ill so that they can stay at home. A clear sign of faked illness is when a child complains of stomach aches or headaches on school days, but is fine at weekends.

School phobia may be caused by anxiety at being separated from the parents. This can be caused by the parents' own over-possessive attitude, or it may be that children are worried about what is happening at home while they are at school. Divorce, family illness or bereavement can all cause such anxiety. If one parent dies or leaves the family home, children can worry about the remaining parent. An intimidating teacher or bullying can also be the cause of school phobia. Many children who refuse to go to school are not lazy or disinterested in their own education but, on the contrary, conscientious students who are fearful of failure.

If your child shows signs of school phobia, be firm about the necessity of going to school, and do not give in to faked illness. Discuss your child's attitude towards school with his or her teacher. If necessary, ask for a referral to an educational psychologist.

If the problem seems to be rooted in a situation at the particular school (as would be the case if your child was being bullied) then consider changing schools altogether. Some anxious children do better in smaller schools, where there tends to be more sense of community. Seek recommendations from other parents, phone other schools and ask to visit, and study the reports published by the Office for Standards in Education (OFSTED).

FIGHTING AND AGGRESSION

Small boys seem to enjoy rough and tumble, and some take longer to grow out of it than others. Such tussles are harmless, even if occasionally they end in tears. As a means of settling disputes, they are

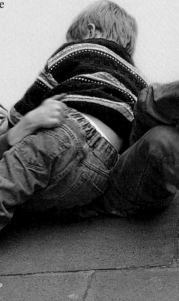

▼ **War games**
Boys love fighting, and banning rough games is practically impossible. But growing boys do not know their own strength and may need to be told where to draw the line between play-fighting and dangerous aggression.

Beating the bullies

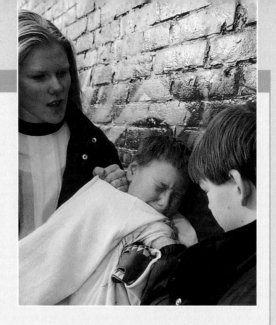

Almost 40 per cent of primary school children say they have been repeatedly bullied, and one in ten say they are both bullies and victims. Persistent bullying can lead to depression and in extreme circumstances even suicide. Some children who fear bullying play truant rather than go to school.

Signs of bullying There are many possible signs when a child is being bullied. Obvious clues include a child coming home from school with damaged clothes or property, unexplained bruises or injuries, or changes in behaviour, such as increased timidity or nervousness around certain children. Other signs of bullying may be a child coming home hungry or asking for extra dinner money, developing a reluctance to go to school, or starting to have eating or sleeping problems.

What to do Make sure your child knows that he or she has your support, and doesn't have to deal with the problem alone. Don't tell him or her to hit back. Encourage your child to tell a teacher and report every act of bullying. Or see the teacher yourself, but make sure you remain calm.

Many children now have mobile phones and bullying by way of phone calls or text messaging is an increasing problem in schools. If your child is a victim of this kind of bullying, tell him or her to write down what the text or caller says and keep a diary of incidents. Consider telling the police as well as a teacher. Making anonymous or abusive phone calls is a criminal offence – contact the charity Bullying Online (www.bullying.co.uk) for further advice.

When your child is the bully Take time to talk to your child and listen to his or her point of view. Be gentle but make it clear that the bullying has to stop – it can be helpful to ask the child what help he or she needs to stop the behaviour. Try to get to the root of any underlying causes – children may start bullying as a response to unhappiness at home or as an attempt to avoid being bullied themselves.

probably no worse than the strategy of withholding friendship, which is common in girls.

Children of school age should be able to control their anger, and express it verbally, not physically. Aggressive children may be copying violent behaviour in the family: if a parent hits out when angry, the child will see this as acceptable.

Aggression in children can be the result of witnessing violence on television. It may also be due to frustration or unhappiness or a reaction to inconsistent discipline. If a child seems always to be fighting, channel the exuberance into energetic games or sports. Aggressive behaviour can sometimes be countered by giving more praise when due, and by arranging activities that require sharing, cooperation and helpfulness.

HELP WITH PROBLEM BEHAVIOUR
If you are worried about your child's behaviour, consult a GP. If your child is aged under five years, your doctor may refer you to a community child psychologist or a child guidance clinic, where you will see a child psychologist or child psychotherapist. In some cases, family therapy may be recommended. A family therapist will look at how family dynamics are affecting the child's behaviour. For this to work, all members of the family must agree to take part in the discussions that form part of the therapy.

Difficult behaviour may stem from a learning disorder or other medical problem. A vision or hearing problem, attention-deficit or hyperactivity disorder (see **ADHD**), **learning difficulties, Asperger's syndrome** and **autism** can have associated behaviour problems. Learning and hearing difficulties are often diagnosed during child development reviews. If you missed these or the problem developed later, contact your doctor or the school health service for an assessment.
SEE ALSO *Adolescence; Child care; Counselling; Parenting; Psychiatry; Psychiatric disorders; Psychoanalysis; Psychotherapy*

CONTACT **Kidscape** 2 Grosvenor Gardens, London SW1W 0DH (020) 7730 3300 (www.kidscape.org.uk)
Parentline Plus helpline 0808 800 2222 (www.parentlineplus.org.uk)
ChildLine Freepost 1111, London N1 OBR; children's helpline 0800 1111 (www.childline.org.uk)
Anti Bullying Campaign (020) 7378 1446
Bullying Online (www.bullying.co.uk)

Acknowledgments

The Reader's Digest Complete A–Z of Medicine and Health was published by the Reader's Digest Association Ltd, London. It was commissioned, edited, designed and typeset by Librios Publishing, 21 Catherine Street, London WC2B 5JS (email: bookcreation@librios.com)

FOR LIBRIOS PUBLISHING

PROJECT MANAGER	Finny Fox-Davies
DESIGN MANAGER	Justina Leitão; Stefan Morris
SENIOR DESIGNERS	Keith Miller; Beatriz Waller
EDITORIAL ASSISTANT	David Popey
EDITORS	Liz Clasen; Antonella Collaro; Celia Coyne; Kim Davies; Henrietta Heald; Jude Ledger; Sam Merrell; Marion Moisy; Charles Phillips
DESIGN ASSISTANTS	Elisa Merino Cuesta; Anthony Morgan; Austin Taylor
PICTURE RESEARCH	Elizabeth Loving
INDEXER	Marie Lorimer
PUBLISHING DIRECTOR	Hal Robinson
EDITORIAL DIRECTOR	Ali Moore
ART DIRECTOR	Peter Laws

FOR THE READER'S DIGEST

COMMISSIONING EDITOR	Jonathan Bastable
ART EDITORS	Louise Turpin; Joanna Walker
PRE-PRESS ACCOUNT MANAGER	Penny Grose
EDITORIAL ASSISTANT	Lucy Murray

READER'S DIGEST GENERAL BOOKS

EDITORIAL DIRECTOR	Cortina Butler
MANAGING EDITOR	Alastair Holmes
ART DIRECTOR	Nick Clark
DEVELOPMENT EDITOR	Ruth Binney
SERIES EDITOR	Christine Noble

CONTRIBUTORS

Elizabeth Adlam MA; Harriet Ainley BSc; Susan Aldridge MSc PhD; Dr Michael Apple BA MBChB MRCGP; Toni Battison RGN RSCN PgDip; Glenda Baum MSc MCSP SRP; Nikki Bradford; Dr Sarah Brewer MA MB BChir; Pat Broad; Dr Harry Brown MBChB DRCOG MRCGP; Jenny Bryan BSc; Rita Carter; Dr Alex Clarke DPsych MSc BSc AFBPsS; Drew Clode BA; Geraldine Cooney BA; Dr John Cormack BDS MB BS MRCS LRCP; Dr Christine Fenn BSc PhD; Dr Vincent Forte BA MB BS MRCGP MSc DA; Dr Judith Hall BSc PhD MBPS; William Harvey BSc MCOptom; Caroline Holland BA; John Isitt BA; Dr Gillian Jenkins BM DRCOG DFFP BA; Georgina Kenyon BA; Dr Laurence Knott BSc MB BS; Dr Jim Lawrie MBBS FRCGP MA (Oxon) MBE; Dr Patricia Macnair MA MBChB Dip Aneasth; Oona Mashta BA; Sheena Meredith MB BS MRCS (Eng) LRCP (Lond); Denise Mortimore BSc PhD DHD; Dr Ian Morton BSc PhD MIBiol; John Newell MA (Camb); Dr Louise Newson BSc MB ChB MRCP MRCGP; Nigel Perryman; Jim Pollard BA MA PCGE; Dr Ann Robinson MBBS MRCGP DCH DRCOG; Dr Christina Scott-Moncrieff MB ChB FFHom; Helen Spence BA; Dr Jenny Sutcliffe PhD MB BS MCSP; Jane Symons; June Thompson RN RM RGV; Helen Varley BA; Patsy Wescott BA; Ann Whitehead MB BS MRCS LRCP MFFP; Dr Melanie Wynne-Jones MB ChB MRCGP DRCOG

CONSULTANTS & ORGANIZATIONS

Alcohol Concern; Alzheimer's Society; Dr Keith Andrews MD FRCP, The Royal Hospital for Neuro-disability; Arterial Disease Clinic; Association of British Insurers; Association for Postnatal Illness; BackCare; Toni Battison RGN RSCN PgDip; Blood Pressure Association; British Dental Health Foundation – Dr Nigel L. Carter BDS LDS (RCS); British Dyslexia Association; British Lung Foundation; British Red Cross; Cancer Research UK; Candle Project – St Christopher's Hospice; Dr A Cann, University of Leicester; Chartered Institute of Environmental Health; CJD Support Network – Alzheimer's Society; Charles Collins MA ChM FRCS Ed – Member of Council for the Royal College of Surgeons of England; Dr Carol Cooper MA MB BChir MRCP; Cystic Fibrosis Trust; Mr R D Daniel BSc FRCS FRCOphth DO; Mr Dai Davies FRCS (plas); Department of Health – Public Awareness; Diabetes UK; Down's Syndrome Association; DrugScope; Eating Disorders Association; The Eyecare Trust; Family Planning Association; Food Standards Agency; Dr Vincent Forte BA MB BS MRCGP MSc DA; Professor Anthony Frew MA MD FRCP; Dr Judith Hall BSc PhD MBPS; International Glaucoma Association; Dr Rod Jaques DRCOG RCGP Dip. Sports Med. (Dist.); Dr Laurence Knott BSc MB BS; Dr Richard Long MD FRCP; Dr John Lucocq MB BCh BSc PhD; Mr W.A. Macleod MBChB FRCSE; Pamela Mason BSc PhD MRPharmS; ME Association; Meningitis Research Foundation; Migraine Action Association; Ian Morton BSc PhD MIBiol; Motor Neurone Disease Association; Multiple Sclerosis Society; National Addiction Centre; National Asthma Campaign; National Autistic Society; National Blood Service; National Eczema Society; National Hospital for Neurology and Neurosurgery; National Kidney Research Fund; National Society for the Prevention of Cruelty to Children; Pituitary Foundation; RADAR (The Royal Association for Disability and Rehabilitation); RELATE; Dr Ann Robinson MBBS MRCGP DCH DRCOG; Royal College of Anaesthetists; Royal College of Speech and Language Therapists; Royal National Institute for Deaf People; Royal National Institute of the Blind; Royal Society for the Prevention of Accidents; Society for Endocrinology; The Society of Chiropodists and Podiatrists and Emma Supple FCPodS; SCOPE; Speakability; Penny Stanway MB BS; Terrence Higgins Trust; Dr Mark Westwood MA(Oxon) MRCP

ILLUSTRATORS

Antony Cobb Associates; Ian Atkinson; Joanna Cameron @ Antony Cobb; Michael Courtney; Chris Forsey; Kevin Jones Associates; Andrew Laws; Katie Laws; Keith Miller; Michael Saunders; Beatriz Waller; Martin Woodward

PICTURE CREDITS

l=left, *r*=right, *t*=top, *b*=bottom, *c*=centre, *a*=above, *bw*=below
Bubbles: Chris Rout 75, 79; Bruno Zarbi 84; Jonathon Chappell 95; Loisjoy Thurston 101*b*; Nikki Gibbs 116; Lucy Tizzard 136; Frans Rombout 137 & 141; Lupe Cunha 140; Vicky Bonomo 156; Anthony Dawton 158. **Corbis:** 132. **Getty Stone:** 103. **Angela Hampton Family Life Picture Library:** 70. **London Scientific Films/Oxford Scientific Films** 93*t*; 107*b*. Courtesy of **The Meningitis Research Foundation** 28*b*. **Medipics:** 25*c*; 76; 94; 101*tc*; 125*t*; MIG: 26*b*; 32*b*; 151; MII: Harry Przekop 93*c*; Ellen Harmon 104, 111. **Photofusion:** Paul Baldesare 159. **Rainbow:** Mark Gibson 80; Jeff Greenberg 82; Dan McCoy 106. **Science Photo Library:** BSIP; LA/Filin.Herrera 64; Saturn Stills 98; Sheila Terry 72; John Eastcott & Yva Momatiuk 107*t*; BSIP, Gounot 135, 142; Astrid & Hans-Frieder Michler 143; Dr P Marazzi 145. **Rex Features:** 85, 99. **Studio photography** John Freeman 66, 86, 91*b*, 125*b*, 146-147, 154. **Viewing Medicine:** 15*t*, 25*t*, 27*t*, 27*c*, 28*t*, 30*ba*, 31*b*, 32*t*, 32*ba*, 44-49, 77, 160. **Wellcome Photo Library:** 15*b*, 25*b*-26*t*, 26*ca*, 26*c*, 26*cbw*, 27*ca*, 27*cbw*, 27*b*, 28*tbw* & 28*ba*, 29*t*-29*c*, 29*b*, 30*t*, 30*tbw*, 30*b*-31*tbw*, 31*ba*, 32*tbw*, 33-37*t*, 37*b*, 39*t*, 39*b*, 41*t*, 41*b*, 81. John Wildgoose 87, 89-91*t*, 92, 93*b*, 96, 101*t*, 101*bc*, 102, 107*c*, 109, 123.

The **Symptom sorter** in this book is based on 'Symptom Sorter' by Dr Vincent Forte and Dr Keith Hopcraft (Radcliffe Medical Press).